Ultrasonic Periodontal Debridement

ULTRASONIC PERIODONTAL DEBRIDEMENT

Theory and Technique

Marie D. George

Adjunct Faculty
University of Pittsburgh School of Dental Medicine, Pittsburgh, PA
Community College of Philadelphia, USA

Timothy G. Donley

Private Practice, Periodontics & Implantology, Bowling Green, KY
Adjunct Professor, Dental Hygiene, Western Kentucky University, USA

Philip M. Preshaw

Professor of Periodontology
School of Dental Sciences and Institute of Cellular Medicine
Newcastle University, UK

WILEY Blackwell

Editorial offices
1606 Golden Aspen Drive, Suites 103 and 104, Ames, Iowa 50010, USA
The Atrium, Southern Gate, Chichester, West Sussex, PO19 8SQ, UK
9600 Garsington Road, Oxford, OX4 2DQ, UK

For details of our global editorial offices, for customer services and for information about how to apply for permission to reuse the copyright material in this book please see our website at www.wiley.com/wiley-blackwell.

Library of Congress Cataloging-in-Publication Data

George, Marie D. (Marie Diane), 1962- author.
  Ultrasonic periodontal debridement : theory and technique / Marie D. George, Philip M. Preshaw, Timothy G. Donley.
    p. ; cm.
  Includes bibliographical references and index.
  ISBN 978-1-118-29545-8 (pbk.)
  I. Donley, Timothy G. (Timothy Gerard), 1959- author. II. Preshaw, Philip, author. III. Title.
  [DNLM: 1. Periodontal Debridement – instrumentation. 2. Periodontal Debridement – methods.
3. Periodontitis – therapy. 4. Ultrasonic Therapy – instrumentation. 5. Ultrasonic Therapy – methods. WU 242]
  RK361
  617.6'32 – dc23

                                                                                          2014000624

A catalogue record for this book is available from the British Library.

Cover image: Cover photos taken by Ali Seyedain, DMD, MDS and Daniel Bair, DMD, MDS, University of Pittsburgh School of Dental Medicine, Department of Periodontics.

Typeset in 10/12pt TimesLTStd by Laserwords Private Limited, Chennai, India
Printed and bound in Singapore by Markono Print Media Pte Ltd

3 2018

Contents

About the Authors

Marie D. George, RDH, MS

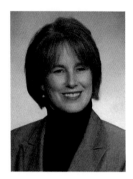

Marie D. George is a clinician, author, and educator, with current appointments as an Adjunct Instructor in the Department of Dental Hygiene at both the University of Pittsburgh School of Dental Medicine and the Community College of Philadelphia. Her past appointments at the University of Pittsburgh include Assistant Professor of Dental Hygiene and Clinical Research Coordinator in the Department of Periodontics. She received a Bachelor of Science Degree in Dental Hygiene from West Liberty State College (now West Liberty University) and a Master of Science Degree in Dental Hygiene from West Virginia University, where she was a two-time recipient of the Procter and Gamble/ADHA Institute for Oral Health Fellowship. She has developed and presented evidence-based educational programs specific to ultrasonic instrumentation to dental hygiene students, pre- and post-doctoral dental students and faculty, and practicing clinicians, nationally and internationally.

Timothy G. Donley, DDS, MSD

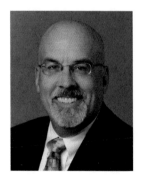

Timothy G. Donley is currently in the private practice of Periodontics and Implantology in Bowling Green, KY and is an Adjunct Professor in the College of Health and Human Services at Western Kentucky University. After graduating from the University of Notre Dame, Georgetown University School of Dentistry, and completing a general practice residency, he practiced general dentistry. He then returned to Indiana University where he received a Master of Science Degree in Periodontics. He has published numerous articles in peer-reviewed journals. He lectures throughout the world on topics of interest to clinical hygienists and dentists.

Phillip M. Preshaw, BDS, FDS RCSEd, FDS (Rest Dent) RCSEd, PhD

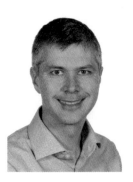

Philip M. Preshaw is Professor of Periodontology at Newcastle University, United Kingdom. He received his Dental Degree from the University of Newcastle in 1991 and his PhD in 1997. He is a registered specialist in Periodontics and is a Fellow of the Royal College of Surgeons of Edinburgh. His main research interests are investigations of the pathogenesis of periodontal disease, and links between diabetes and periodontal disease. Professor Preshaw lectures frequently, and has numerous publications in peer-reviewed scientific journals. He has been awarded a UK National Institute of Health Research (NIHR) National Clinician Scientist Fellowship, a Distinguished Scientist Award from the International Association for Dental Research, and a King James IV Professorship from the Royal College of Surgeons of Edinburgh.

Foreword

In periodontics, a notable paradigm shift occurred in the late 1980s when scientific evidence began to clearly indicate that the host response to the microbial challenge, and not the oral microbes and their end-products themselves, was responsible for periodontal destruction. This opened a new era in our profession – one in which understanding and controlling the host response became of paramount importance. We are now in the midst of another shift – one that directly affects the non-surgical approach to periodontal treatment by focusing on biofilm disruption and conservation of tooth structure rather than calculus and cementum removal. How fitting that this book, *Ultrasonic Periodontal Debridement: Theory and Technique*, has been written to address the rationale and techniques for implementing this new paradigm into practice. Organized and written in a practical way, the content will resonate with all clinicians engaged in helping patients control their periodontal disease. Written by Marie George, RDH, MS; Timothy Donley, DDS, MSD; and Philip Preshaw, BDS, FDS, RCSEd, PhD, this book provides evidence-based data from clinical studies which support the fundamental instrumentation principles and techniques that are described. The authors bring their combined years of experience in dental hygiene education, periodontal practice, and periodontal academia to provide the reader with a sound guide to the use of ultrasonics as the primary treatment modality in periodontal debridement. As a trained dental hygienist and periodontist engaged in academic dentistry, I found this book to be the most thorough resource on ultrasonic debridement I have read.

The book is organized into three sections. Section I focuses on foundational knowledge. In this section, the authors provide a historical and literature-based perspective on the evolving paradigm of the etiology and pathogenesis of periodontal disease. They further describe how the evolution of our understanding of the disease process should now lead to an evolution in how we treat our patients. To support this concept, the authors provide a thorough review of the evidence on the effectiveness of ultrasonic versus hand instruments in removing the plaque biofilm and calculus, and the efficacy of these two instrumentation techniques in resolving the clinical manifestations of disease. Overall, this section provides the scientific evidence and rationale for the current paradigm shift away from scaling and root planing (SRP) with hand instruments to biofilm disruption and deposit removal using ultrasonic debridement.

Section II focuses on sonic and ultrasonic scaling technology and techniques. It includes the principles of ultrasonic transduction, oscillation, and mechanisms of action (mechanical, irrigation, cavitation, and acoustic microstreaming). The authors move on to provide a review of operational variables critical to ultrasonic debridement that includes operating frequency, power setting, and water flow rate. Evidence of the impact of each of these variables on the disruption of the plaque biofilm, removal of calculus, and damage to the root surface is provided. A comprehensive discussion of ultrasonic tip design and selection, along with a description of the clinical consequences of improper selection, complete this section. Excellent tables and figures are provided that augment the technical descriptions in the text.

Section III provides the practical clinical application of the information from the first two sections. A review of patient assessment and the role of clinical parameters in determining the diagnosis and treatment needs are included. Also included is a review of the relationship among pocket anatomy, deposit type, and tooth anatomy, and instrument selection. This section closes with detailed information on the fundamental principles and techniques of ultrasonic instrumentation. It is an excellent resource for the practitioner wanting in-depth understanding of the principles and techniques for ultrasonic instrumentation and the ideal strategies for instrument sequencing. It contains a wealth of clinical "how to" images depicting exactly what should be done by tooth and by area of the mouth, supplemented with details on tip selection and instrumentation techniques for advanced furcation defects and implants.

Finally, three case studies are included to provide further details on how to approach the decision-making process and, ultimately, the rationale for selecting ultrasonic debridement as the treatment of choice for non-surgical periodontal therapy. The case studies comprise a patient description, clinical photographs, and clinical charting and radiographs as well as excellent descriptions and clinical images depicting instrument selection and placement. The level of detail in the descriptors and images in this section and throughout this book sets it apart from others that cover periodontal instrumentation techniques.

Throughout this book, authors George, Donley, and Preshaw provide a framework for making evidence-based, non-surgical therapeutic decisions when treating patients with periodontal disease. As stated in the book "It is clear that over the last few decades, our understanding of periodontal pathogenesis and microbiology has advanced significantly, and it is important to now interpret this information in the context of the clinical situation to help us decide upon the best treatment strategies for our patients." I sincerely believe that all who read this book will find it to be their "go to" evidence-based resource on the theory, rationale, and technique for the effective use of ultrasonic debridement in providing periodontal therapy to their patients.

Karen F. Novak, D.D.S., M.S., Ph.D.
Professor, Department of Periodontics
& Dental Hygiene
Associate Dean for Professional Development
& Faculty Affairs
University of Texas Health Science Center at
Houston School of Dentistry

Preface

The purpose of this book is to provide the reader with clear, evidence-based guidance in the practicalities of periodontal ultrasonic instrumentation. The material is organized as a guide that the clinician can follow, and commences with the theory of ultrasonic debridement therapy, followed by detailed, precise instruction in ultrasonic instrumentation technique, and concludes with a series of case studies of real-life clinical scenarios.

Why is such a book needed? After all, there are many excellent textbooks on periodontology currently available. However, a surprising finding is that little attention is paid to the principles of ultrasonic therapy in most periodontology textbooks, certainly much less than is devoted to the intricacies of manual instrumentation or periodontal surgical techniques. Yet, the ultrasonic scaler is one of the instruments most frequently used by dental clinicians worldwide.

This book is aimed at all clinicians who treat patients with periodontal diseases, students (both dental students and dental hygienist students), dental residents, general dentists, dental hygienists, and periodontists. It is intended to be a resource that all dental clinicians can utilize to improve their understanding of why ultrasonic debridement therapy is the core treatment strategy for managing periodontitis, and the practicalities of how to do it.

The publication of this book is very timely as today's dental professionals find themselves in the midst of a paradigm shift in terms of the best way to provide periodontal treatment. In previous decades, periodontal treatment had focused on calculus and cementum removal as the primary end-points of periodontal therapy; this was the scaling and root planing (SRP) era. However, modern understanding of the processes and therapeutic strategies in the treatment of periodontal disease has shifted the approach that is used in non-surgical periodontal therapy away from SRP to a treatment modality that is focused on biofilm disruption and conservation of tooth structure; this is the concept of periodontal debridement therapy, and is the topic of this book.

Accordingly, the approach to clinical instrumentation is also changing, and the standard of care is shifting from a manual instrumentation approach (which met the objectives of SRP therapy) to ultrasonic instrumentation, which meets the objectives of periodontal debridement therapy.

Many clinicians, however, still remain unsure about how exactly they should perform ultrasonic debridement, and often mistakenly apply the principles of manual instrumentation to ultrasonic instruments. The instruction and development of manual instrumentation skills continue to predominate in dental and dental hygiene educational programs. Many clinical curricula for students of dental and dental hygiene include an unwarranted prerequisite for demonstrated competency in hand instrumentation before exposure to ultrasonic instrumentation, which perpetuates the inappropriate application of manual instrumentation techniques to ultrasonic instruments. Yet, ultrasonic instruments are completely different from manual instruments, and should be used in a completely different way.

Historically, there has been a lack of comprehensive instructional resources specific to ultrasonic instrumentation. The objective of this textbook is to meet this need by providing the faculty and students with a core text to facilitate the practical instruction of ultrasonic instrumentation theory and technique, and align curricula to the current, evidence-based treatment concept of periodontal debridement. The book is also very relevant for dental clinicians at all stages of their career and training who wish to improve their knowledge of ultrasonic debridement techniques.

Marie D. George
Timothy G. Donley
Philip M. Preshaw

Acknowledgments

The content of this book is founded on the work of scientists, researchers, engineers, and clinicians, including those cited within and others less recognized, whose expertise and accomplishments are responsible for the advancements made in periodontal science and ultrasonic technology. We value your contributions and hope this book does your work justice.

We acknowledge the creativity and skill of our photographers and illustrators: Daniel Bair, DMD, University of Pittsburgh School of Dental Medicine, Department of Periodontics – clinical photography; Robert Benton, RDB Imaging, LLC, Dover, PA – typodont and equipment photography; Thomas Robbins, graphic illustrator, York, PA; and Tyler Webster, graphic artist, Bowling Green, KY.

We are grateful to Mike Gregory and Kilgore International, Inc. for providing the typodonts utilized to demonstrate technique; Patricia Parker and Hu-Friedy Mfg. Co. LLC, for providing the scaling unit and tips used clinically; and Jonathan Krizner, DDS, for the use of his dental office.

Our thanks to the team at John Wiley & Sons, particularly Rick Blanchette, Melissa Wahl, and Teri Jensen, for the guidance, support, and patience extended throughout this process.

Last but not least, we wish to extend heartfelt gratitude to our families and friends, especially *Jennifer George*, and *Kelly, Kevin, Connor and Cara Donley*, who have accommodated us throughout the writing process, for without their support, this book may have never come to fruition.

Marie D. George
Timothy G. Donley
Philip M. Preshaw

About the Companion Website

This book is accompanied by a companion website:

www.wiley.com/go/george/ultrasonic

The website includes:

- Powerpoints of all figures from the book for downloading
- PDFs of tables from the book

SECTION 1

FOUNDATIONAL CONCEPTS

Chapter 1

The treatment of periodontal disease: the shift from "SRP" to "Periodontal Debridement"

CHAPTER OBJECTIVES

1. To provide a historical perspective regarding the development of instrumentation concepts in periodontal therapy.
2. To consider the historical focus on endotoxin, and how this led to the preeminence of root planing as a treatment strategy to remove calculus and cementum.
3. To consider the role of the plaque biofilm in driving periodontal inflammation, and the importance of the inflammatory host response in periodontal tissue breakdown.
4. To explain the current understanding of periodontal pathogenesis and periodontal microbiology, and how this has informed the development of modern periodontal treatment strategies.
5. To review the evidence that supports the paradigm shift away from root planing (a damaging form of periodontal therapy) to periodontal debridement therapy (root surface debridement), which achieves the aims of biofilm disruption and removal while at the same time preserving cementum.

Periodontal disease is not new. Archeological investigations have revealed evidence of alveolar bone loss affecting human remains dating from around 700,000 years ago (Dentino et al., 2013). Descriptions of conditions that we would now refer to as periodontitis can be found in a number of ancient textbooks, papyruses, and manuscripts, such as *al-Tasrif*, the medical encyclopedia written by Albucasis (936–1013) in Moorish Spain. This document was translated into Latin during the twelfth century, and was one of the primary medical texts used in European universities until the seventeenth century (Shklar and Carranza, 2012). In addition to describing the clinical features of periodontitis, some of these early authors also described treatment strategies for the condition. For example, Albucasis focused on the role of calculus in the disease process, and his works included depictions of a variety of instruments for the removal of calculus that bear a striking similarity to many of the periodontal instruments still being used today (Figure 1.1).

Over the centuries, and more specifically, over recent decades, our understanding of periodontal diseases has evolved exponentially, and as a result, so have the treatment strategies that we employ to manage the condition. Therefore, we no longer treat periodontitis by washing the mouth with wine and water, as advocated by

Ultrasonic Periodontal Debridement: Theory and Technique, First Edition. Marie D. George, Timothy G. Donley and Philip M. Preshaw.
© 2014 John Wiley & Sons, Inc. Published 2014 by John Wiley & Sons, Inc.

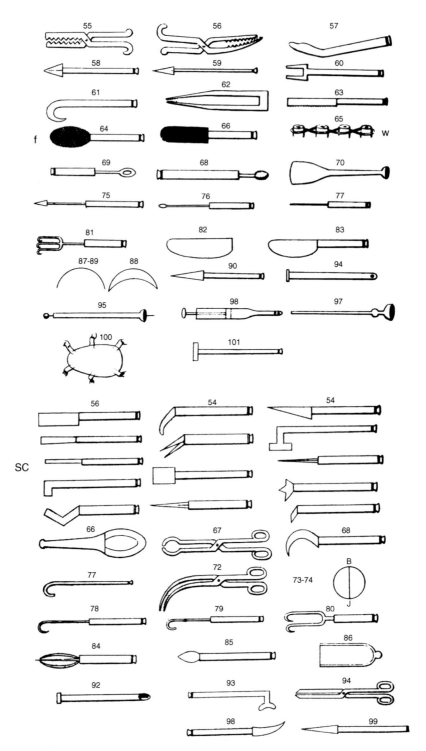

Figure 1.1 Illustration of Albucasis' periodontal instruments. Note the instruments recognizable as (SC) scalers (left side, halfway down), as well as (f) files (top left, 4th instrument down), blades and scissors, and (w) wiring for mobile teeth (top right, 4th illustration down). (*Source*: Carranza, 2012. Reproduced with permission of Elsevier)

Fauchard (1678–1761), the "father of modern dentistry," in his 1728 dentistry textbook *Le Chirurgien Dentiste*. To help us decide which treatment methods are the most appropriate for modern day clinicians to utilize, it is important to briefly review the scientific advances that have been made in periodontology, as these have greatly influenced the treatment protocols that have been used in clinical practice over recent years.

EARLY CONCEPTS OF THE PATHOGENESIS OF PERIODONTAL DISEASE

Calculus the irritant

If we spend a moment to imagine the likely oral health status of many of the people living in the Middle Ages, in the time of Albucasis, for example, we would probably conjure up images of abundant calculus deposits, inflamed gingival tissues, gingival bleeding, and halitosis. It is understandable that these early dentists focused on the role of calculus "accretions" as the cause of the problem, and developed methods for trying to remove the deposits. The etiological role of calculus in the pathogenesis of periodontal disease was unquestioned for many centuries. In the United States of America, Riggs (1810–1885) regarded calculus as the cause of periodontal disease, and treated the condition by the meticulous removal of calculus from pockets, "curettage" of the soft tissues, and oral hygiene instruction (Dentino et al., 2013). For many years, periodontal disease was referred to as "Riggs' Disease"; such was the influence of this pioneering clinician.

The emergence of microbiology as a discipline, coupled with improvements in microscopy, led to studies of the bacterial composition of dental plaque. The term "pyorrhea alveolaris" was introduced in the late nineteenth century to denote conditions in which gingival pockets

developed, which permitted bacteria to "infect and destroy" the periodontal tissues and the alveolar bone. During this era, the importance of local factors in the etiology of periodontal disease was unquestioned, and calculus was viewed as being directly responsible for the tissue damage that was observed in patients with periodontitis. This concept led directly to the emergence of treatment strategies that focused exclusively on calculus removal as the endpoint of periodontal therapy.

The role of plaque

The etiological role of plaque in the development of gingival inflammation was confirmed in experimental studies on gingivitis conducted in the 1960s: upon cessation of oral hygiene practices over periods of 3–4 weeks, plaque accumulation resulted in gingivitis, which was reversed following plaque removal and resumption of normal oral hygiene (Loe and Silness, 1963; Loe et al., 1965). These studies were revolutionary in that they moved the focus of attention away from calculus and more toward plaque as the predominant etiological factor of periodontal diseases.

But how did plaque "cause" periodontal disease? The *nonspecific plaque hypothesis* made the assumption that periodontal disease (as well as caries) resulted from the production and release of harmful substances from the entire plaque mass. Inherent to this theory were the suppositions (i) that there must be a threshold for these substances (above which periodontal disease will develop, and below which it will not), and (ii) that the amount of plaque present is the main determinant of risk for disease. In other words, this theory suggests that the more plaque a patient has, the more periodontal disease he/she will have. But any clinician knows that this does not hold true; some patients have very poor oral hygiene and lots of plaque, but do not develop advanced periodontitis, and conversely, some patients with good oral hygiene and minimal plaque levels can develop advanced disease.

Further microbiological investigations led to the emergence of the *specific plaque hypothesis* (Loesche, 1976). This theory held that only certain types of plaque cause disease, because they contain specific bacteria that are particularly pathogenic; for example, they release irritants such as endotoxin, H_2S, lactic acid, and bacterial collagenase, which cause injury to the periodontal tissues. It is noteworthy that both the nonspecific and the specific plaque hypotheses considered periodontal tissue breakdown to result from a direct effect of harmful substances released from the plaque bacteria.

Endotoxin

The term "*endotoxin*" was originally introduced to denote toxic substances within bacterial cells that were released upon death of the bacteria. Today, the term is used synonymously with the term "*lipopolysaccharide*" (LPS), which is a component of the outer cell wall of gram-negative bacteria. LPS consists of a polysaccharide chain linked covalently to a lipid moiety, and it is essential for maintaining the structural integrity of the bacterial cell wall. LPS induces strong immune and inflammatory responses in higher order species such as humans and other animals, which is why it is so important in the pathogenesis of a number of diseases, including periodontal disease. LPS invokes strong immune–inflammatory responses precisely because it is present in gram-negative bacteria; higher order species have evolved to be able to detect and respond to LPS because it signals the presence of such bacteria.

Research in the 1960s and 1970s identified that endotoxin was present in the outer surfaces of cementum in teeth affected by periodontitis (Daly et al., 1980). It was hypothesized that this endotoxin would limit the effectiveness of periodontal therapy, because even if plaque and calculus were removed from the root surface, the endotoxin still present in the cementum would continue to irritate the tissues and thus compromise healing following treatment. This presumption led to the preeminence of the treatment concept known as "root planing," often combined as a treatment strategy with scaling, and abbreviated as "SRP" ("*scaling and root planing*").

SCALING AND ROOT PLANING (SRP)

SRP became established as a periodontal treatment concept because of the prevailing belief that calculus, endotoxin, and necrotic cementum needed to be removed from the root surface. Necrotic cementum was considered to be that part of the cementum (the outer layer) that was impregnated with endotoxin from the overlying plaque mass. *Root planing* was therefore employed to vigorously remove this outer layer of cementum by heavy-duty planing of the root surface (think about planing a door to make it fit the door frame better).

What were the objectives of SRP?

We firstly need to decide what is meant by SRP, which actually refers to two separate treatment techniques, "scaling" and "root planing." Root planing was described as a treatment procedure in the early parts of the twentieth century (Hartzell, 1913; Stillman, 1917) and since then, there have been many different definitions of scaling and root planing in the periodontal literature over the decades. In the 1953 edition of Glickman's *Clinical Periodontology* textbook, the use of scalers is described to remove calculus deposits and to "smooth the tooth surface" by the removal of "softened, necrotic cementum" (Glickman, 1953). Root planing is not mentioned at all, but another treatment strategy, "curettage," is. Curettage was described as the "management of the inner surface of the soft tissue wall" of the pocket, in which the epithelial lining of the pocket was forcibly removed to create a bleeding connective tissue surface against the tooth root, which was believed at that time to result in better healing. This was often achieved by applying pressure to the outside of the pocket (i.e., the free gingiva) with a finger while performing the upstroke with a curet located in the pocket, so that the pocket epithelium was forcibly stripped off. The inner blade of the curet would be removing plaque/calculus/cementum on the upstroke while the outer blade would be stripping off the epithelial lining of the pocket. However, curettage has not been employed for many years, because of the pain it can cause, and also because it was later shown that outcomes following SRP with curettage were the same as those following SRP alone (Echeverria and Caffesse, 1983). Coupled with the confusion that different definitions can create is the further complication that root planing is often accomplished using instruments called curets, and the term "curettage" has sometimes been used interchangeably with the term "root planing." Curettage is no longer undertaken, and will not be discussed further in this book.

Glickman's 1953 textbook has evolved over the years, with the most recent version being the 11th edition (2012), now entitled *Carranza's Clinical Periodontology*. In that book, *scaling* is defined as "the process by which biofilm and calculus are removed from both supragingival and subgingival tooth surfaces, but no deliberate attempt is made to remove tooth substance along with the calculus." *Root planing* is defined as "the process by which residual embedded calculus and portions of cementum are removed from the roots to produce a smooth, hard, clean surface" (Pattison and Pattison, 2012). In order to clarify matters, our interpretations of these various terms are presented in Box 1.1. Confusion is created, however, by other interpretations and definitions of these terms that are commonly used (Box 1.2 and Box 1.3). In broad terms, and for the purpose of this book, we consider that

the objective of scaling is the removal of supra- and subgingival calculus (without damaging the tooth surface), and the objective of root planing is the removal of subgingival calculus together with superficial layers of cementum.

Box 1.1: Periodontal treatment terminology as utilized in this book

Scaling Instrumentation performed to remove/reduce calculus deposits, both supragingival and subgingival, and without damaging the tooth surface

Root planing Instrumentation performed to remove subgingival calculus and also cementum (and thereby endotoxin) from the root surface

Curettage Instrumentation performed to remove the soft tissue lining of the periodontal pocket

Root surface debridement Instrumentation performed to disrupt and remove the subgingival biofilm, and to remove calculus, but without intentional removal of cementum

---

Box 1.2: MeSH terms that describe periodontal treatments

MeSH terms

MeSH terms are *Medical Subject Headings* – they are a series of definitions created by the United States National Library of Medicine (NLM) that are used for indexing journal articles and books.

MeSH terms in relation to periodontal treatment include:

Dental scaling

Removal of dental plaque and dental calculus from the surface of a tooth, from the surface of a tooth apical to the gingival margin accumulated in periodontal pockets, or from the surface

Box 1.2 *(continued)*

coronal to the gingival margin (Year introduced: 1991, updated from 1972).

Root planing

A procedure for smoothing of the roughened root surface or cementum of a tooth after subgingival curettage or scaling, as part of periodontal therapy (Year introduced: 1992).

Subgingival curettage

Removal of degenerated and necrotic epithelium and underlying connective tissue of a periodontal pocket in an effort to convert a chronic ulcerated wound to an acute surgical wound, thereby insuring wound healing and attachment or epithelial adhesion, and shrinkage of the marginal gingiva (Year introduced: 1965).

Periodontal debridement

Removal or disruption of dental deposits and plaque-retentive dental calculus from tooth surfaces and within the periodontal pocket space without deliberate removal of cementum as done in root planing and often in dental scaling. The goal is to conserve dental cementum to help maintain or re-establish a healthy periodontal environment and eliminate periodontitis by using light instrumentation strokes and nonsurgical techniques (e.g., ultrasonic, laser instruments) (Year introduced: 2011).

Authors' comments

These terms fit reasonably well with modern interpretations. The MeSH definitions of *dental scaling* and *periodontal debridement* are closely aligned with our understanding of scaling and root surface debridement as presented in Box 1.1. Importantly, the MeSH definition of *periodontal debridement* emphasizes that cementum is not deliberately removed, and, importantly, this distinguishes the procedure from *root planing*. By simply referring to smoothing of roughened surfaces, the MeSH definition for *root planing* does not adequately convey the damaging nature of the procedure. Clearly, *subgingival curettage* is an outdated treatment modality.

These terms were taken from the National Center for Biotechnology Information website: NCBI. National Center for Biotechnology Information MeSH Terms [Internet]. 2013 [cited 2013 June 14]. Available from: http://www.ncbi.nlm.nih.gov/mesh/

Box 1.3: ADA Code on Dental Procedures and Nomenclature (CDT) that describes periodontal treatments

CDT Codes

CDT Codes are defined by the American Dental Association and are used by dentists and insurance companies in the United States for coding dental treatments.

CDT Codes in relation to periodontal treatment include:

D4341 and D4342 periodontal scaling and root planing

This procedure involves instrumentation of the crown and root surfaces of the teeth to remove plaque and calculus from these surfaces. It is indicated for patients with periodontal disease and is therapeutic, not prophylactic, in nature. Root planing is the definitive procedure designed for the removal of cementum and dentin that is rough, and/or permeated by calculus or contaminated with toxins or microorganisms. Some soft tissue removal occurs. This procedure may be used as a definitive treatment in some stages of periodontal disease and/or as a part of presurgical procedures in others.

(D4341 is used if there are ≥ 4 teeth per quadrant to treat, and D4342 is used if there are < 4 teeth per quadrant to treat).

D4355 full mouth debridement to enable comprehensive evaluation and diagnosis

The gross removal of plaque and calculus that interfere with the ability of the dentist to perform a comprehensive oral evaluation. This preliminary procedure does not preclude the need for additional procedures.

Box 1.3 (continued)

Authors' comments

The description of *root planing* presented here is consistent with the aim of removing cementum, dentine, and calculus that defines this treatment procedure. The description also acknowledges that both hard and soft tissue damage results. The emphasis on removing toxins (i.e., endotoxin) is not consistent with modern understanding of (i) microbial biofilms, (ii) the fact that endotoxin is loosely adherent to cementum, or (iii) periodontal pathogenesis. The description of *full mouth debridement* here refers to a procedure for removing gross plaque and calculus deposits to enable a complete oral examination. This interpretation is at variance with the modern understanding of the term *debridement* as shown in Box 1.1. Clearly, the CDT codes will result in most practitioners undertaking periodontal therapy that is destructive to the root surface.

These terms were taken from the CDT Codes published by the ADA: American Dental Association Code on Dental Procedures and Nomenclature 2012 (effective for the calendar year 01 January 2013 through 31 December 2013).

The (historical) justification for root planing

Given the historical belief that calculus was the primary etiology of periodontitis, it is understandable that treatment strategies focused on the complete removal of all calculus. As mandated in 1953, "every speck of it must be removed" (Glickman, 1953). To the modern clinician, calculus is certainly plaque retentive and unsightly, and removing it is an important part of therapy; but, is it really possible to remove every speck of it? A number of studies have addressed this issue. In a study of 690 root surfaces in 11 patients with moderate/advanced periodontitis, the percentage of surfaces with residual calculus following instrumentation with a sonic scaler was 32%, with manual instruments was 27%, and with both instruments used together was 17% (Gellin et al., 1986). The researchers also found that deeper pockets were associated with more residual calculus following instrumentation. In another study, 476 surfaces on 101 extracted teeth were instrumented using both ultrasonic and hand instruments. Following the instrumentation, 19% of surfaces had residual calculus that could be detected clinically, and 57% of surfaces had residual calculus on examination under the microscope (Sherman et al., 1990). In a study of 21 patients requiring multiple extractions, SRP was provided prior to the extractions and the percentage of the subgingival surfaces that were free of calculus was determined with a stereomicroscope (Caffesse et al., 1986). In pockets that were 4–6 mm deep, only 43% of surfaces were free of calculus after closed SRP, and in pockets that were > 6 mm deep, only 32% of surfaces were free of calculus after treatment. The extent of residual calculus was directly correlated with probing depth, and was greatest at the cemento–enamel junction, and in association with grooves and in furcations (Caffesse et al., 1986)

Taken collectively, the outcomes from a number of similar studies that have investigated this issue confirm that nonsurgical instrumentation is effective in significantly reducing the amount of calculus on root surfaces. However, complete calculus removal is not usually achieved, and deeper pockets are more likely to harbor residual calculus following treatment, with anywhere from approximately 3% to 80% of instrumented root surfaces showing some residual calculus after instrumentation (Claffey et al., 2004).

Furthermore, we clinicians are not very effective in determining whether we have fully removed calculus or not (Figure 1.2). For example, in the study described above, there was a high false-negative response rate in that 77% of the surfaces that were determined to have residual calculus when examined under the microscope had been clinically scored previously

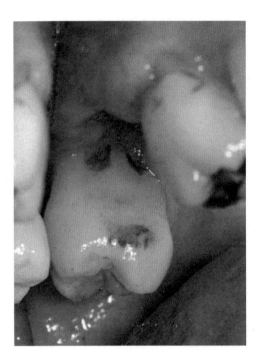

Figure 1.2 Residual calculus that had been missed during previous periodontal instrumentation. This patient had received previous full mouth periodontal instrumentation on several occasions and was in the maintenance phase of therapy. Tooth #14 (FDI 26) was extracted because of endodontic problems, and as the extraction site healed, the tissues at the mesial aspect of #15 (FDI 27) receded to reveal subgingival calculus that had not been removed by the prior periodontal instrumentation (dark brown areas in two locations close to the gingival margin)

as being free of calculus (Sherman et al., 1990). This underscores the difficulties of determining the thoroughness of subgingival instrumentation. Calculus detection is technically very challenging due to the complex anatomy of the pocket environment. While supragingival calculus can be identified by direct vision and drying of the tissues, subgingival calculus is much more difficult to identify, unless the deposits are very large and can be detected by a periodontal probe or calculus explorer, or can be seen at the pocket opening. Radiographic detection of calculus is similarly unreliable; a sensitivity for radiographic detection of calculus of only 44% has been reported (i.e., only 44% of surfaces known to have calculus present clinically could be detected on radiographic examination) (Buchanan et al., 1987).

Besides calculus removal, the other main rationale that has been given for planing the roots is removal of cementum as the means by which to remove endotoxin (sometimes described as the removal of "contaminated cementum"). Early investigators reported that endotoxin was present in the cementum of teeth affected by periodontitis and that it was biologically active with an inhibitory effect on cellular function (Aleo et al., 1974). Further studies reported that fibroblasts did not attach to periodontally compromised roots until after the cementum was removed, or the endotoxin was removed chemically (Aleo et al., 1975; Assad et al., 1987). These studies implied that for periodontal treatment to be successful, there needs to be meticulous removal of cementum and endotoxin from the root surfaces. Further justification for this approach came from studies that showed that planing the roots resulted in significant reductions in the amount of endotoxin present, typically rendering the root surfaces nearly free of endotoxin (Jones and O'Leary, 1978). It was considered that removing the endotoxin creates a root surface that is more "biologically acceptable," or more "compatible with wound healing," though this concept has rarely been defined in a clinical context (most studies that investigated the impact of endotoxin removal were laboratory-based studies that investigated, e.g., colonization of root surfaces by fibroblasts before and after cementum/endotoxin removal). The outcome of these studies was that root planing was considered a beneficial treatment strategy because it resulted in cementum and endotoxin removal, but it was never completely clear as to precisely how much cementum should be removed, or whether excessive cementum removal could have unwanted effects.

Unwanted outcomes of root planing

As already described, root planing has two main aims: (i) removal of subgingival calculus and (ii) removal of the outer layer of cementum (and thereby endotoxin). In order to achieve this, the root surface is planed to remove the outer layers of cementum together with any overlying calculus. The obvious major disadvantage of this treatment modality is that tooth substance (i.e., cementum) is physically removed, and the main consequence of this is dentin sensitivity.

Other disadvantages of root planing are that it can be unpleasant for the patient as a result of the force applied and scraping sensations. Furthermore, root planing has been reported to result in significant duration and magnitude of pain, with many patients self-medicating to relieve the pain (Pihlstrom et al., 1999). Root planing requires the use of local anesthetics, can take a long time to perform (raising concerns about cost effectiveness), and can be tiring (for both the patient and the clinician).

How much cementum is removed during root planing depends on many factors, such as the sharpness of the instrument, the adaptation of the instrument to the root surface, the number of strokes used, and the lateral force applied. The issue of tooth substance removal when using manual or ultrasonic instruments is discussed in more detail in Chapter 2. What constitutes a clinically acceptable amount of tooth surface removal during periodontal instrumentation is difficult to define. However, it has been suggested that a defect depth of 0.5 mm (i.e., a total cumulative removal of 0.5 mm of cementum) over 10 years (e.g., in a patient undergoing long-term periodontal maintenance care) is clinically acceptable (Flemmig et al., 1997; Flemmig et al., 1998a; Flemmig et al., 1998b). On this basis, and assuming that the same root surfaces are instrumented each year, cementum removal per year should not exceed 50 μm (i.e., 0.05 mm per year, in other words 1/20th of a millimeter per year). If we assume one episode of instrumentation per year on each surface, this suggests that a single episode of instrumentation should not remove more than 50 μm of cementum. If there were four episodes of instrumentation per year for supportive periodontal therapy, this suggests that each episode of maintenance instrumentation should not remove more than

12.5 μm of cementum to remain within the 50 μm per year limit. While this concept is theoretically interesting to consider, it must be borne in mind, of course, that it is actually impossible to quantify the depth of cementum removal that may be occurring during any particular root planing episode.

Taken to an extreme, root planing would result in the removal of all cementum from a root surface (Figure 1.3). Achieving this could have significant negative impacts in terms of root sensitivity, but was once considered a desirable aim of treatment (the removal of all "diseased cementum" was a treatment end-point). It would only be possible to test whether there are any clinical benefits of complete cementum removal by achieving direct vision onto the root surface following reflection of a periodontal flap. This concept was first tested in an experimental periodontitis study in dogs in which an open surgical approach was utilized for root planing

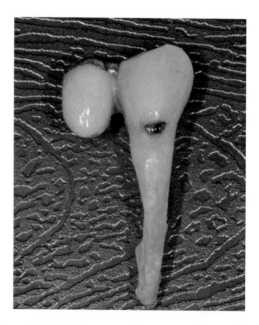

Figure 1.3 This lower premolar was an abutment for a cantilever bridge and was extracted as a result of progression of periodontitis, severe mobility and sensitivity. The patient underwent many courses of root planing, which has resulted in the removal of all the cementum and much of the dentine at the distal aspect of the root, with subsequent pulpal involvement. (Image courtesy of Dr. Ian Dunn, Liverpool, UK)

(Nyman et al., 1986). In test quadrants, all the cementum was planed from the root surfaces, whereas in control quadrants, the roots were polished with rubber cups and polishing paste. After 2 months, histological assessment indicated that healing was similar in all quadrants, whether or not the cementum had been removed. It was concluded that the removal of root cementum with the purpose of eliminating endotoxin does not seem to be necessary for achieving healing following therapy.

The same research design was then applied in a human study of 11 patients treated surgically using a split mouth design. In two quadrants, teeth were root planed to remove all calculus and all cementum while in the other two quadrants, only calculus was removed (Nyman et al., 1988). The patients were monitored for 24 months, and the outcomes of treatment (probing depth reductions and attachment gains) were similar following both treatment modalities, suggesting that there was no benefit of complete cementum removal. This led the authors to further question the prevailing dogma that "infected" root cementum should be removed by root planing (Nyman et al., 1988).

CURRENT CONCEPTS OF PERIODONTAL PATHOGENESIS

Some of the most significant research that has influenced our understanding of periodontal pathogenesis was conducted in Sri Lanka, an island nation in the Indian Ocean. A population of 480 male laborers working in two tea plantations underwent periodontal assessment at regular intervals over a 15-year period (Loe et al., 1986). These individuals had no access to dental care, and had not received any periodontal treatment at any point in their lifetime. The participants did not follow any conventional oral hygiene measures and, as a result, had uniformly abundant plaque and calculus deposits throughout the dentition. Yet, despite the fact that plaque and calculus were present in large quantities in all

the participants, they did not all have periodontitis. In fact, the population could be subdivided into three groups: (i) those with rapid progression of periodontal disease (approximately 10% of the total population), (ii) those with moderate progression (~80%), and (iii) those with no progression of periodontal disease beyond gingivitis (~10%). The annual rate of disease progression varied between 0.1 mm and 1.0 mm in the rapid progression group, and between 0.05 mm and 0.5 mm in the moderate progression group. This study confirmed that not all people are equally susceptible to periodontitis, despite the fact that plaque bacteria are ubiquitously present. This finding has underpinned our current understanding of periodontal pathogenesis and continues to influence our approach to treatment.

Biofilm: The driver of periodontal inflammation

Dental plaque is more accurately described as a biofilm. *Biofilms* are composed of microbial cells (e.g., bacteria) encased within a matrix of extracellular polymeric substances such as polysaccharides, proteins and nucleic acids (Teughels et al., 2012). Biofilm structures vary according to the environmental conditions, but several features are common to most biofilms. For example, water channels are present, which remove waste products and bring fresh nutrients to the deeper layers of the film. Surface structures such as fronds dissipate the energy of fluid flowing over the biofilm (and thereby protect against mechanical shearing forces). Microcolonies of bacteria may exist at discreet areas of the biofilm according to the local environment, and steep chemical gradients (e.g., in oxygen or pH) can exist, which create distinct microenvironments.

The formation of the plaque biofilm can be divided into three phases: (i) formation of pellicle on the tooth surface, (ii) initial attachment of bacteria, and (iii) the colonization/maturation phase. *Pellicle* (usually referred to as acquired pellicle) is an organic material that coats all hard and soft surfaces in the oral cavity. It contains a large variety of peptides, proteins, and glyco-proteins that can function as adhesion sites for bacteria. The initial attachment of bacteria to the pellicle commences within minutes, and the primary colonizers (i.e., those bacteria which adhere to the pellicle first) are typically those which possess surface "adhesin" molecules that allow them to attach to the pellicle. These include *Streptococcus* species, which form 60–80% of the bacteria present within the first 4–8 hours, as well as *Haemophilus, Neisseria, Actinomyces,* and *Veillonella* species. These primary colonizers provide new binding sites for adhesion by other bacteria which themselves could not attach to the pellicle. Furthermore, the metabolic activity of these primary colonizers affects the local environment. For example, the primary colonizers utilize oxygen, which results in low oxygen tension locally that permits the survival of more anaerobic bacterial species.

The accumulation of primary colonizing bacteria creates binding sites for other bacteria (the secondary colonizers) to attach, in a process called "coadhesion." The biofilm is now maturing and increasing in complexity as multiple species colonize and adhere to bacteria present in the plaque mass. Some of the key secondary colonizers include *Prevotella intermedia, Fusobacterium nucleatum, Porphyromonas gingivalis, Prevotella loescheii,* and *Capnocytophaga* species. As the biofilm matures, there is a shift in the microbial population from primarily gram-positive organisms to anaerobic gram-negative species.

The biofilm is, therefore, a complex environment of multiple bacterial species cohabiting within the "slime" matrix that the bacteria produce (Marsh, 2005). The major nutrient sources for the bacteria present in the biofilm are the saliva and the gingival crevicular fluid (GCF). There are also many metabolic relationships between bacteria in the biofilm, in which waste products from certain species are utilized as nutrients by other species. For example, metabolic byproducts such as succinate from

Capnocytophaga ochracea and protoheme from *Campylobacter rectus* enhance the growth of *P. gingivalis.* Communication between bacteria also occurs within the biofilm, a process known as quorum sensing. For example, bacteria may secrete a signaling molecule that accumulates locally and triggers a response such as the expression of specific genes once a certain threshold is reached. This may occur only when a certain cell density has been reached; in other words, when the bacteria sense that the bacterial population has reached a critical mass, or quorum.

As our knowledge of the nature of the plaque biofilm has increased, this has forced researchers to re-evaluate previously held beliefs about the role of plaque in the etiology of periodontal disease. For example, earlier in this chapter, the *nonspecific plaque hypothesis* was described, in which it was believed that periodontal disease resulted from the release of noxious products from the entire plaque mass, with the inherent assumption that the more plaque a person has, the more periodontal disease they will have. But, this clearly does not fit with our clinical observations of patients, or the studies of tea laborers in Sri Lanka (Loe et al., 1986). This theory was replaced with the *specific plaque hypothesis*, which considered that only certain plaque is pathogenic, depending on the presence of specific microorganisms that produce substances that result in direct tissue damage (Loesche, 1976). This concept gained favor as researchers identified that the composition of subgingival plaque was different in healthy as opposed to diseased sites, and a large number of studies were conducted to try to identify the microbiota that could distinguish periodontal disease from health (Socransky and Haffajee, 1992). Cluster analyses identified that certain species were much more commonly found in advanced periodontitis, such as *P. gingivalis, Tannerella forsythia,* and *Treponema denticola,* which were described as the "red complex" of species, associated with deep pocketing (Socransky et al., 1998). However, it was never clear if these organisms *caused* the

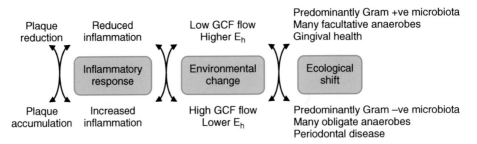

Figure 1.4 The Ecologic Plaque Hypothesis. Accumulation of plaque results in inflammation in the gingival tissues (gingivitis) and other environmental changes that favor the growth of gram-negative species. In turn, the inflammatory response alters the environment (e.g., increased GCF flow, altered redox potential) which can favor the growth of certain species associated with periodontitis (i.e., an ecological shift occurs). GCF, gingival crevicular fluid; E_h, redox potential; Gram +ve, Gram-positive; G−ve, Gram-negative. (Adapted from Marsh, 1994)

disease (i.e., were responsible for the tissue damage leading to the formation of a deep pocket), or just *correlated* with it (i.e., were particularly well suited to living in the environment of a deep pocket). Even as these studies were being conducted, it was beginning to be recognized that specific species (pathogens) are necessary, but by themselves are insufficient, for disease to occur – the host response also plays a role.

Our current understanding of the role of the plaque biofilm in periodontal disease is captured in the *ecologic plaque hypothesis* (Marsh, 1994). This theory holds that both the total amount of dental plaque and the specific microbial composition of plaque may contribute to the progression of periodontitis. In health, the biofilm composition is relatively stable, in a state of dynamic equilibrium (or "microbial homeostasis"), and in balance with a steady-state low level immune/inflammatory response. Changes to this steady state may result from any perturbations of the host response, such as brought about by a (nonspecific) increase in the accumulation of plaque, or changes in host factors (e.g., changes in hormone levels such as those occurring during pregnancy), or changes in environmental factors (e.g., smoking, stress, diet). As inflammation develops in the tissues, GCF flow increases, which may favor the growth of certain species that utilize GCF constituents as a nutrient source. Tissue degradation, increased GCF

flow and inflammation all could result in a shift in the microbial population, potentially favoring the growth of the predominantly anaerobic pathogenic species that have been associated with advanced periodontal disease (Figure 1.4).

Endotoxin is loosely adherent to the cementum

Studies commencing in the 1970s indicated that LPS from gram-negative bacteria was so firmly attached to the root surface, and considered to have such a negative effect on the potential for healing following therapy, that extensive cementum removal was advocated in the form of root planing (Aleo et al., 1974; Aleo et al., 1975; Assad et al., 1987). Cementum that contained LPS was considered to be "infected," "necrotic" or "contaminated," and the traditional treatment model held that removal of the outer layer (or indeed all) of the cementum by root planing, as the means by which to remove endotoxin, was necessary to achieve periodontal health (Jones and O'Leary, 1978; O'Leary, 1986).

However, a number of studies reported contrasting evidence, which resulted in questions being asked about the necessity for root planing teeth in order to remove endotoxin. For example, it was identified that endotoxin did not penetrate significantly into the cementum (it was located at the surface), and most of the LPS identified on roots was associated with tooth deposits and bacteria on the root surface (Hughes and Smales, 1986; Hughes et al., 1988; Hughes and Smales, 1990; Ito et al., 1985). Furthermore, studies of extracted teeth indicated that LPS was superficially (i.e., loosely) bound, and could be removed by brushing, leading to the suggestion that systematic root planing to remove cementum was not indicated. For example, in a study of teeth that had been extracted because of advanced periodontal disease, it was identified that 39% of the LPS present in the cementum could be removed by gentle washing in water for 1 minute and 60% could be removed by brushing for 1 minute (Moore et al., 1986). In other words, 99% of the LPS was removed by comparatively gentle procedures. Subsequent studies confirmed that as few as 15 strokes with a hand instrument resulted in significant reductions in the quantity of endotoxin within root surfaces, suggesting that extensive root planing was not warranted as a periodontal treatment strategy (Cheetham et al., 1988). The concept that LPS should be regarded as being *associated* with cementum, rather than being *bound* to cementum, was further supported by research on extracted teeth that were immersed in LPS for periods of 2–12 weeks. The researchers identified that LPS adhered to the surfaces only (whether teeth were healthy or had been periodontally involved) and did not penetrate into the cementum, and that the binding of LPS to the root surfaces was weak (Nakib et al., 1982).

To summarize, while it has been clearly established that LPS is present in cementum of periodontally involved teeth (Maidwell-Smith et al., 1987; Wilson et al., 1986), the great majority of the LPS is located at the cementum surface, and is mainly associated with the subgingival biofilm, rather than being firmly bound to the cementum itself. LPS that is present can be removed by gentle techniques such as washing with water or polishing the root surface, and therefore extensive root planing in order to remove LPS cannot be justified.

Periodontitis is an inflammatory disease

As we have learned, periodontitis was historically thought to result from tissue damage caused directly by noxious products released from bacteria in plaque, but we now know that the majority of the tissue breakdown results from the inflammatory response to the biofilm. In other words, the host response is the major determinant of how much tissue breakdown occurs. Current thinking about the nature of periodontitis is captured in these statements taken from the periodontal literature:

> "Periodontitis is more accurately categorized as a nonresolving inflammation that is ineffective in eliminating the initiating pathogens, and that is sustained by the same"
>
> (Chapple 2009).

> "Periodontitis is an inflammatory disease initiated by oral microbial biofilm … it is the host response to the biofilm that destroys the periodontium"
>
> (Van Dyke 2008).

The recognition that the inflammatory response is responsible for the majority of tissue breakdown helps to explain why some people are more susceptible to periodontitis (even if they have good oral hygiene), why periodontitis can seem to run in families (because aspects of immune and inflammatory responses can be genetically determined), and why some people appear to be relatively resistant to developing periodontitis, despite the fact that they might have very poor plaque control.

Evidence of inflammation can be identified even in clinically healthy tissues, with a continuous (but low) flow of GCF, and migration of small numbers of neutrophils from the gingival capillaries through the tissues to the sulcus. As plaque accumulation increases (or other environmental changes occur), the clinical signs of gingivitis develop in parallel with histological changes such as increased vascular permeability and vasodilatation, increased GCF flow, and increased infiltration of the tissues by leukocytes, particularly neutrophils and lymphocytes. Macroscopically, the tissues become red and swollen as a result of increased blood flow and increased permeability of the vessels, allowing fluid (and cells) to accumulate. As the inflammation becomes more established, there is accumulation of inflammatory cells in the connective tissues, increased release of matrix metalloproteinases (MMPs) and lysosomal contents from neutrophils, collagen destruction (resulting in collagen-depleted areas), and apical migration of the junctional epithelium in order to maintain an intact epithelial barrier. As the area of inflammation extends deeper into the underlying connective tissues, alveolar bone resorption commences to protect the bone, which "retreats" from the advancing inflammatory front. Thus, the clinical signs of periodontitis are evident as a result of breakdown of collagen fibers in the gingival connective tissue and periodontal ligament, apical migration of the junctional epithelium (resulting in the pocket becoming deeper) and alveolar bone resorption. A complex network of cytokines, destructive enzymes and other inflammatory mediators plays a key role in the inflammatory processes, and it is believed that excessive, prolonged, and dysregulated inflammatory responses are responsible for the majority of the tissue damage that we observe in our patients (Kinane et al., 2011; Preshaw and Taylor, 2011). Some people are more susceptible to periodontitis than others, and it is likely that these individuals have a more aggressive (or up-regulated) inflammatory response to the bacterial challenge. Unfortunately, we do not, as yet, have a reliable method for identifying these individuals.

It was previously believed that periodontitis progressed at a slow, steady continuous rate throughout life, which might vary in different populations (Loe et al., 1978). However, this did not fit easily with the later observations that identified different rates of progression of disease in the Sri Lankan tea laborer population (Loe et al., 1986). Further studies established that the disease appeared to progress at different rates within an individual, with episodes of more rapid tissue breakdown ("bursts" of disease activity), alternating with periods of periodontal stability (Haffajee and Socransky, 1986; Socransky et al., 1984). These two contrasting theories of disease progression were known as the *linear progression theory* and the *random burst theory* of periodontal disease progression. Modern multilevel modeling statistical techniques have essentially combined the linear progression and random burst theories to suggest that both are probably manifestations of the same phenomenon, namely, that some sites improve while others progress in a cyclical manner (Gilthorpe et al., 2003).

PERIODONTAL DEBRIDEMENT THERAPY

It is clear that over the last few decades, our understanding of periodontal pathogenesis and microbiology has advanced significantly, and it is important to now interpret this information in the context of the clinical situation to help us decide on the best treatment strategies for our patients. Periodontal inflammation is initiated and perpetuated by the subgingival biofilm, and it is the inflammatory response that causes the majority of tissue breakdown that results in the clinical signs and symptoms of periodontitis. The cyclical manner of disease progression highlights the importance of regarding periodontal therapy as a life-long commitment to controlling periodontal inflammation, something which we must explain to all of our patients. We must utilize plaque control (by the patient) and biofilm disruption via instrumentation (by the clinician) as the vehicles by which to reduce periodontal inflammation and thereby promote a stabilization of the periodontal tissues. Resolution of inflammation results in shrinkage of the inflamed tissues, leading to reductions in probing depths (so pockets are easier to keep clean). Reductions in probing depths will also result in environmental changes in the pocket environment which favor less pathogenic species, as explained by the ecologic plaque hypothesis (Figure 1.4). The question must be asked as to what is the best method of providing periodontal instrumentation, and to answer that question, we must first consider what the objectives of instrumentation are.

The objectives of modern periodontal debridement must fit with our current understanding of periodontal disease processes, and include

- disruption and removal of the subgingival biofilm;
- removal of plaque-retentive factors such as calculus;
- conservation of tooth structure;
- creation of a biologically acceptable root surface; and
- resolution of inflammation.

These objectives are considered in more detail in Box 1.4. In broad terms, the overall aim of periodontal treatment is resolution of inflammation, because continued chronic inflammation in the periodontal tissues results in the tissue damage that we recognize as periodontitis. Plaque control by the patient and disruption of the biofilm by the clinician remain the cornerstones of periodontal therapy. The subgingival biofilm initiates and perpetuates the chronic inflammatory response in the periodontal tissues, and therefore biofilm reduction/removal should result in a reduction in inflammation. Changes in the quantity and quality of the biofilm following instrumentation, and resultant reductions in inflammation both will have the effect of altering the local environment in the periodontal pocket, and as the gingival tissues shrink (resolution of inflammation), the pockets will become shallower, and therefore easier to maintain (by both patient and clinician), as well as also favoring the growth of less pathogenic species in the subgingival environment.

Box 1.4: Objectives of modern periodontal debridement

Disruption and removal of the sub-gingival biofilm

The subgingival biofilm initiates and perpetuates the chronic inflammatory response in the periodontal tissues. It is the host response against the bacterial challenge which causes the majority of the tissue breakdown that characterises periodontitis. The host response is frustrated, however, in attempts to deal with the bacterial challenge because the bacteria are effectively outside the body (notwithstanding that they are in the pocket, in the oral cavity). The bacteria can never be fully eradicated, and their continued presence drives the inflammatory response. Treatment should aim to disrupt the biofilm, and remove as much of it as is possible (while accepting that it is impossible to remove all of the bacteria). The aim of reducing the bacterial challenge is to effect a reduction in inflammation, which will have clinical benefits (shallower pockets are easier to maintain) and will also alter the pocket environment favouring less pathogenic species.

Removal of plaque-retentive factors such as calculus

Calculus does not cause periodontal disease. However, it is unsightly and plaque-retentive, and therefore should be removed. It is not possible to remove all the calculus, however, and complete calculus removal should not be the aim of treatment.

Conservation of tooth structure

Excessive removal of tooth structure can result in sensitivity, and gouges in the root surface from periodontal instruments can be plaque-retentive. Modern instrumentation techniques should therefore cause minimal damage to the root surface and should conserve tooth structure. This is particularly important given that we know that periodontal maintenance care is a life-long enterprise, and patients with periodontitis may undergo multiple episodes of periodontal instrumentation over their lifetime.

Box 1.4 (continued)

Creation of a biologically acceptable root surface

This is quite hard to define, but basically means that the root surface post-instrumentation should not hinder resolution of inflammation. For example, it should be reasonably smooth, and free of plaque-retentive factors (such as obvious pieces of calculus). We do not need to focus on trying to remove endotoxin (as we now know that it is removed from root surfaces very easily – see text) because it is removed almost as a by-product of modern instrumentation techniques, contributing further to the concept of creating a biologically acceptable root surface.

Resolution of inflammation

The overall aim of periodontal debridement is resolution of inflammation, and that is achieved by the objectives outlined above, together with optimal plaque control by the patient.

The objectives of periodontal debridement listed in Box 1.4 would not be achieved by root planing (which has the objectives of removal of calculus and cementum/endotoxin). Furthermore, the requirement for cementum removal was questioned by the research conducted by Nyman and colleagues, who demonstrated using open surgical approaches to root surface instrumentation, that simply polishing the root surfaces resulted in equivalent treatment outcomes to those obtained following complete removal of all calculus and cementum from the roots, both in an animal model (Nyman et al., 1986) and in human studies (Nyman et al., 1988). The realization that LPS does not penetrate deeply into the cementum, and is only loosely retained on root surfaces led to a paradigm shift in treatment concepts for periodontitis. This approach was pioneered by Kieser's research group who introduced the term *root surface debridement* (RSD) to indicate a light-touch, gentler form of instrumentation to promote plaque removal, yet with preservation of cementum (Moore et al., 1986, Smart et al., 1990). This treatment approach seemed to fit well with the use of ultrasonic instruments which, as

a result of their biophysical properties (discussed later in this book), could be utilized to facilitate biofilm disruption and endotoxin flushing, but with the preservation of cementum.

In a study of periodontally compromised extracted teeth that were free of visible calculus, ultrasonic debridement applied with a force of approximately 50 g for a mean time of 78 seconds (s) per root utilizing an overlapping "cross-hatching" instrumentation technique resulted in a reduction of LPS to levels that were similar to those found in healthy, nonperiodontally compromised, control teeth (Smart et al., 1990). The expended time of 78 s per root equated to instrumenting for $0.8\,\text{s/mm}^2$ of root surface. Later work by the same group revealed that even in the presence of calculus deposits, the use of ultrasonic instruments with light pressure and overlapping strokes resulted in mean reductions in LPS content per tooth from 1900–29,200 ng prior to instrumentation to <22 ng post-instrumentation (for comparison, LPS levels at nonperiodontally involved control teeth ranged from 15 to 28 ng) (Chiew et al., 1991). These reductions in LPS levels occurred despite the fact that not all the calculus was removed by the instrumentation procedure (planimetric assessment revealed that the mean percentage coverage of the roots by visible calculus was 74% before debridement and 34% after). The authors concluded that the therapeutic benefits of periodontal instrumentation are derived from the removal of plaque rather than cementum or calculus.

Kieser proposed that periodontal therapy should be performed in a pragmatic, staged approach, adopting a RSD methodology (as opposed to root planing) that involves the use of periodontal instruments at light pressures, with multiple overlapping strokes, the aim being to remove plaque and, at the same time, to minimize removal of cementum. It would not be possible to assess the success of such a treatment strategy by simply trying to identify whether calculus had been removed or not, or whether root surfaces were "smooth" or "rough," or "soft" or "hard."

Table 1.1 Key differences between Then (*scaling and root planing*) and Now (*root surface debridement*)

THEN: *we had SRP*	NOW: *we have RSD*
In "those days," the nonsurgical treatment strategy was SRP (scaling and root planing) ... why was this?	Modern understanding of the disease process indicates that RSD (root surface debridement) is the treatment of choice... why is this?
Answer: Calculus was regarded as *the* etiological factor in periodontal disease, and therefore, every effort should be made to remove it.	*Answer:* Periodontal disease results from a complex interplay between the bacterial biofilm and the host immune-inflammatory response. Calculus does not cause disease (though it is plaque-retentive).
And: Research seemed to suggest that endotoxin was embedded in the cementum, therefore, surface layers of cementum should be removed too.	*And:* It has been shown clearly that endotoxin is only loosely adherent to cementum; therefore there is no need to try to remove cementum. Furthermore, cementum removal is damaging to the root surface and results in problems of pain and sensitivity (particularly if done repeatedly over the years).
The upshot of this: There was an emphasis on using sharp, bladed instruments to try to remove calculus and cementum and smooth the root surface.	*The upshot of this:* Ultrasonic instruments are indicated to debride the root surface, that is, to disrupt and reduce the biofilm, and remove calculus, but without causing intentional removal of cementum. This is a gentler, less destructive form of treatment that achieves the same clinical outcomes, but without causing tissue damage. It is also more time efficient, and appropriate for use year-on-year in a typical periodontal maintenance patient.

Indeed, as previously demonstrated, complete calculus removal is not an achievable outcome or a realistic target of treatment, and clinicians are notoriously poor at identifying whether or not calculus has been removed. Instead, the outcome of RSD must be determined by assessing the soft tissue response following therapy. The biological response to the treatment should be the main measure of the success of therapy, in other words, whether inflammation has reduced. Kieser advocated that probing depths should be measured at 3 months following therapy, and for sites which continued to demonstrate bleeding on probing, further instrumentation could be performed. By utilizing ultrasonic instruments, this treatment model would permit multiple episodes of instrumentation to remove plaque (or disrupt and reduce the biofilm, as we would now say), to maximize the likelihood of resolution of inflammation, but without causing extensive tissue damage or cementum removal. In other words, it was suggested that RSD should aim to disrupt and remove plaque from periodontally involved root surfaces (rather than removing part of the root surface itself), and the success of therapy should be assessed on the basis of the healing response (Corbet et al., 1993).

Patients with periodontitis typically will cycle through episodes of more intensive instrumentation, separated by longer periods of periodontal maintenance care. The treatment philosophies advocated by Kieser et al. fit well with this "biological model" of periodontal treatment provision. The response to treatment is assessed by evaluating the soft tissue response, particularly the degree of inflammation (visual assessment as well as evaluation of bleeding on probing), rather than focusing exclusively on the presence of residual calculus. Calculus should be removed, as it is plaque retentive, but calculus removal alone should no longer be considered the end-point of therapy.

Multiple episodes of instrumentation are likely to be experienced by the typical patient with periodontitis during their lifetime; chronic periodontitis is a chronic disease, and its management must be regarded as a chronic (i.e., life-long) process. It is, therefore, important that periodontal debridement is performed in such a way as to avoid damaging the root surface and to conserve root structure, to avoid problems of sensitivity and the creation of plaque-retentive features such as grooves. RSD offers further advantages in this context in that local anesthetic may not be required (in contrast to root planing), and full mouth treatment approaches are much more practical and easier to achieve. An overview of the key differences between scaling/root planing and periodontal debridement is shown in Table 1.1.

Root planing cannot be justified as a treatment concept because (i) it causes unnecessary damage to the root surface, (ii) its target outcome (i.e., calculus and cementum removal) cannot be verified, and, (iii) it is not necessary to plane roots for the purposes of endotoxin removal. Put more simply, it is not possible to remove all the calculus, we do not wish to remove the cementum, and, therefore, root planing does not have a place in modern periodontal therapy.

Instead, we advocate that periodontal debridement therapy (RSD) be utilized as the treatment of choice for nonsurgical periodontal therapy. The desired end-point of treatment is resolution of inflammation, and this is achieved by disrupting the biofilm and reducing the bacterial

challenge. Clinical methods for conducting periodontal debridement therapy are discussed in the next chapter, with a focus on the techniques that achieve the objectives of biofilm disruption and preservation of root cementum.

REFERENCES

Aleo JJ, De Renzis FA, Farber PA, Varboncoeur AP. The presence and biologic activity of cementum-bound endotoxin. *J Periodontol* 1974; 45: 672–5.

Aleo JJ, DeRenzis FA, Farber PA. An *in vitro* attachment of human gingival fibroblasts to root surfaces. *J Periodontol* 1975; 46: 639–45.

Assad DA, Dunlap RM, Weinberg S, Ahl D. Biologic preparation of diseased root surfaces. An in vitro study. *J Periodontol* 1987; 58: 30–3.

Buchanan S, Jenderseck R, Granet M, Kircos L, Chambers D, Robertson PB. Radiographic detection of dental calculus. *J Periodontol* 1987; 58: 747–51.

Caffesse RG, Sweeney PL, Smith BA. Scaling and root planing with and without periodontal flap surgery. *J Clin Periodontol* 1986; 13: 205–10.

Chapple ILC. Periodontal diagnosis and treatment - where does the future lie? *Periodontol 2000* 2009; 51: 9–24.

Cheetham WA, Wilson M, Kieser JB. Root surface debridement--an in vitro assessment. *J Clin Periodontol* 1988; 15: 288–92.

Chiew SYT, Wilson M, Davies EH, Kieser JB. Assessment of ultrasonic debridement of calculus-associated periodontally-involved root surfaces by the limulus amoebocyte lysate assay: an in vitro study. *J Clin Periodontol* 1991; 18: 240–4.

Claffey N, Polyzois I, Ziaka P. An overview of nonsurgical and surgical therapy. *Periodontol 2000* 2004; 36: 35–44.

Corbet EF, Vaughan AJ, Kieser JB. The periodontally-involved root surface. *J Clin Periodontol* 1993; 20: 402–10.

Daly CG, Seymour GJ, Kieser JB. Bacterial endotoxin: a role in chronic inflammatory periodontal disease? *J Oral Pathol* 1980; 9: 1–15.

Dentino A, Lee S, Mailhot J, Hefti AF. Principles of periodontology. *Periodontol 2000* 2013; 61: 16–53.

Echeverria JJ, Caffesse RG. Effects of gingival curettage when performed 1 month after root instrumentation. A biometric evaluation. *J Clin Periodontol* 1983; 10: 277–86.

Flemmig TF, Petersilka GJ, Mehl A, Hickel R, Klaiber B. The effect of working parameters on root substance removal using a piezoelectric ultrasonic scaler in vitro. *J Clin Periodontol* 1998a; 25: 158–63.

Flemmig TF, Petersilka GJ, Mehl A, Hickel R, Klaiber B. Working parameters of a magnetostrictive ultrasonic scaler influencing root substance removal in vitro. *J Periodontol* 1998b; 69: 547–53.

Flemmig TF, Petersilka GJ, Mehl A, Rudiger S, Hickel R, Klaiber B. Working parameters of a sonic scaler influencing root substance removal in vitro. *Clin Oral Investig* 1997; 1: 55–60.

Fogel HM, Pashley DH. Effect of periodontal root planing on dentin permeability. *J Clin Periodontol* 1993; 20: 673–7.

Gellin RG, Miller MC, Javed T, Engler WO, Mishkin DJ. The effectiveness of the Titan-S sonic scaler versus curettes in the removal of subgingival calculus. A human surgical evaluation. *J Periodontol* 1986; 57: 672–80.

Gilthorpe MS, Zamzuri AT, Griffiths GS, Maddick IH, Eaton KA, Johnson NW. Unification of the "burst" and "linear" theories of periodontal disease progression: a multilevel manifestation of the same phenomenon. *J Dent Res* 2003; 82: 200–5.

Glickman I (1953) The scaling and curettage technique for the eradication of the periodontal pocket. In: *Clinical Periodontology*, pp. 716–24. Philadelphia: WB Saunders.

Haffajee AD, Socransky SS. Attachment level changes in destructive periodontal diseases. *J Clin Periodontol* 1986; 13: 461–75.

Hartzell TB. The operative and post-operative treatment of pyorrhea. *Dental Cosmos* 1913; 55: 1094–101.

Hughes FJ, Auger DW, Smales FC. Investigation of the distribution of cementum-associated lipopolysaccharides in periodontal disease by scanning electron microscope immunohistochemistry. *J Periodontal Res* 1988; 23: 100–6.

Hughes FJ, Smales FC. Immunohistochemical investigation of the presence and distribution of cementum-associated lipopolysaccharides in periodontal disease. *J Periodontal Res* 1986; 21: 660–7.

Hughes FJ, Smales FC. The distribution and quantitation of cementum-bound lipopolysaccharide on periodontally diseased root surfaces of human teeth. *Arch Oral Biol* 1990; 35: 295–9.

Ito K, Hindman RE, O'Leary TJ, Kafrawy AH. Determination of the presence of root-bound endotoxin using the local Shwartzman phenomenon (LSP). *J Periodontol* 1985; 56: 8–17.

Jones WA, O'Leary TJ. The effectiveness of in vivo root planing in removing bacterial endotoxin from the roots of periodontally involved teeth. *J Periodontol* 1978; 49: 337–42.

Kinane DF, Preshaw PM, Loos BG. Host-response: understanding the cellular and molecular mechanisms of host-microbial interactions-consensus of the Seventh European Workshop on Periodontology. *J Clin Periodontol* 2011; 38 Suppl 11: 44–8.

Loe H, Anerud A, Boysen H, Morrison E. Natural history of periodontal disease in man. Rapid, moderate and no loss of attachment in Sri Lankan labourers 14 to 46 years of age. *J Clin Periodontol* 1986; 13: 431–40.

Loe H, Anerud A, Boysen H, Smith M. The natural history of periodontal disease in man. The rate of periodontal destruction before 40 years of age. *J Periodontol* 1978; 49: 607–20.

Loe H, Silness J. Periodontal disease in pregnancy I. Prevalence and severity. *Acta Odontol Scand* 1963; 21: 533–51.

Loe H, Theilade E, Jensen SB. Experimental gingivitis in man. *J Periodontol* 1965; 36: 177–87.

Loesche WJ. Chemotherapy of dental plaque infections. *Oral Sci Rev* 1976; 9: 65–107.

Maidwell-Smith M, Wilson M, Kieser JB. Lipopolysaccharide (endotoxin) from individual periodontally involved teeth. *J Clin Periodontol* 1987; 14: 453–6.

Marsh PD. Microbial ecology of dental plaque and its significance in health and disease. *Adv Dent Res* 1994; 8: 263–71.

Marsh PD. Dental plaque: biological significance of a biofilm and community life-style. *J Clin Periodontol* 2005; 32 Suppl 6: 7–15.

Moore J, Wilson M, Kieser JB. The distribution of bacterial lipopolysaccharide (endotoxin) in relation to periodontally involved root surfaces. *J Clin Periodontol* 1986; 13: 748–51.

Nakib NM, Bissada NF, Simmelink JW, Goldstine SN. Endotoxin penetration into root cementum of periodontally healthy and diseased human teeth. *J Periodontol* 1982; 53: 368–78.

Nyman S, Sarhed G, Ericsson I, Gottlow J, Karring T. Role of "diseased" root cementum in healing following treatment of periodontal disease. An experimental study in the dog. *J Periodontal Res* 1986; 21: 496–503.

Nyman S, Westfelt E, Sarhed G, Karring T. Role of "diseased" root cementum in healing following treatment of periodontal disease. A clinical study. *J Clin Periodontol* 1988; 15: 464–8.

O'Leary TJ. The impact of research on scaling and root planing. *J Periodontol* 1986; 57: 69–75.

Pattison AM, Pattison GL (2012) Scaling and root planing. In: *Carranza's Clinical Periodontology*, (eds.) M. G. Newman, H. H. Takei, P. R. Klokkevold and F. A. Carranza, 11th edn, pp. 461–73. St. Louis, Missouri: Elsevier Saunders.

Pihlstrom BL, Hargreaves KM, Bouwsma OJ, Myers WR, Goodale MB, Doyle MJ. Pain after periodontal scaling and root planing. *J Am Dent Assoc* 1999; 130: 801–7.

Preshaw PM, Taylor JJ. How has research into cytokine interactions and their role in driving immune responses impacted our understanding of periodontitis? *J Clin Periodontol* 2011; 38 Suppl 11: 60–84.

Ritz L, Hefti AF, Rateitschak KH. An in vitro investigation on the loss of root substance in scaling with various instruments. *J Clin Periodontol* 1991; 18: 643–7.

Sherman PR, Hutchens LH, Jewson LG, Moriarty JM, Greco GW, McFall WT. The effectiveness of subgingival scaling and root planing. I. Clinical detection of residual calculus. *J Periodontol* 1990; 61: 3–8.

Shklar G, Carranza FA (2012) The historical background of periodontology. In: *Carranza's Clinical Periodontology*, (eds.) M. G. Newman, H. H. Takei, P. R. Klokkevold and F. A. Carranza, pp. 2–11. St. Louis, Missouri: Elsevier Saunders.

Smart GJ, Wilson M, Davies EH, Kieser JB. The assessment of ultrasonic root surface debridement by determination of residual endotoxin levels. *J Clin Periodontol* 1990; 17: 174–8.

Socransky SS, Haffajee AD. The bacterial etiology of destructive periodontal disease: current concepts. *J Periodontol* 1992; 63: 322–31.

Socransky SS, Haffajee AD, Cugini MA, Smith C, Kent RL, Jr., Microbial complexes in subgingival plaque. *J Clin Periodontol* 1998; 25: 134–44.

Socransky SS, Haffajee AD, Goodson JM, Lindhe J. New concepts of destructive periodontal disease. *J Clin Periodontol* 1984; 11: 21–32.

Stillman PR. The management of pyorrhea. *Dental Cosmos* 1917; 59: 405–14.

Teughels W, Quirynen M, Jakubovics NS (2012) Periodontal microbiology. In: *Carranza's Clinical Periodontology*, (eds.) M. G. Newman, H. H. Takei, P. R. Klokkevold and F. A. Carranza, pp. 232–70. St. Louis, Missouri: Elsevier Saunders.

Van Dyke TE. The management of inflammation in periodontal disease. *J Periodontol* 2008; 79: 1601–8.

Vastardis S, Yukna RA, Rice DA, Mercante D. Root surface removal and resultant surface texture with diamond-coated ultrasonic inserts: an in vitro and SEM study. *J Clin Periodontol* 2005; 32: 467–73.

Wilson M, Moore J, Kieser JB. Identity of limulus amoebocyte lysate-active root surface materials from periodontally involved teeth. *J Clin Periodontol* 1986; 13: 743–7.

Zappa U, Smith BA, Simona C, Graf H, Case D, Kim W. Root substance removal by scaling and root planing. *J Periodontol* 1991; 62: 750–4.

Chapter 2

Comparison of periodontal debridement instrumentation modalities

CHAPTER OBJECTIVES

1. To review the available methods of periodontal debridement including the use of manual instrumentation, ultrasonic instrumentation, and laser energy.
2. To review the evidence that compares the potential for manual and ultrasonic instrumentation to remove calculus and biofilm.
3. To review the evidence that compares the potential for manual and ultrasonic instrumentation to reduce probing depth, increase attachment level, and reduce bleeding on probing (BOP).
4. To assess the difference between manual and ultrasonic instrumentation in terms of root surface damage during use.
5. To review the evidence concerning the use of ultrasonic instrumentation during debridement of dental implant surfaces.

We learned in the first chapter that root planing is an outdated concept. In this new age of *root surface debridement*, the goal of periodontal therapy is biofilm disruption and preservation of root cementum. Biofilm disruption can be accomplished by mechanical means (manual instrumentation and/or ultrasonic instrumentation), and laser-generated energy (Rosen, 2001). With the objectives of modern periodontal debridement clearly in mind (Box 2.1), attention should next be focused on the efficacy, advantages, and limitations of available instrumentation techniques to achieve these objectives.

Box 2.1: Objectives of modern periodontal debridement

- Disruption and removal of the subgingival biofilm
- Removal of plaque retentive factors such as calculus
- Conservation of tooth structure
- Creation of a biologically acceptable root surface
- Resolution of inflammation

EFFICACY OF DEPOSIT REMOVAL

As explained in Chapter 1, it is the formation of bacteria into complex biofilms that initiates the host response that results in periodontal breakdown, with the presence of calculus deposits contributing to the retention of plaque. Visible plaque forms when biofilm grows to the point

---

where it is clinically detectable. We also think of calculus in terms of calcified deposits that can be seen or felt. But, the fact is that not all biofilm develops into plaque, not all plaque forms into calculus, and not all of the calculus that forms is clinically detectable.

For the resolution of periodontal disease, the subgingival microbiota and plaque-retentive deposits must be reduced to a level compatible with periodontal health. Admittedly, the level (of reduction) necessary to facilitate disease resolution is likely to differ between patients, as it is dependent on the host immune system and variations in the presence or absence of risk factors associated with periodontal diseases. Therefore, rather than aiming for an unattainable objective of complete removal of all deposits, an instrumentation method that can predictably remove as much clinically evident and microscopic etiology as possible should be used to insure that an adequate reduction is achieved in all individuals.

Calculus removal

While a number of studies confirm that nonsurgical instrumentation is effective in significantly reducing the amount of calculus on root surfaces, complete calculus removal is not usually achieved (Chapter 1). Comparisons between studies assessing the ability for manual or ultrasonic instrumentation to remove calculus are difficult to make owing to the inability to standardize the characteristics of deposit being removed, the methodology used to remove it, or even the detection of calculus itself before or after therapy. With these limitations in mind, it is not surprising that there is no complete agreement on the calculus removal abilities of different methods of instrumentation (Cobb, 1996). However, most studies suggest that ultrasonic instrumentation removes calculus to a degree similar to that removed via manual instrumentation (Hunter et al., 1984; Breininger et al., 1987; Kepic et al., 1990; Thornton and Garnick, 1992; Apatzidou and Kinane, 2010). One such study of 60 teeth

slated for extraction was undertaken in part to identify and quantify the residual deposits on instrumented root surfaces. Two molar and two nonmolar tooth groups (of 15 teeth each) were alternately treated *in vivo* by manual instrumentation either with a variety of curettes or an ultrasonic instrument. Instrumented and control teeth were then extracted, stained, and analyzed via stereomicroscopy using a calibrated grid. Both manual and ultrasonic instrumentation as performed in this study were equally effective in calculus removal. It is noteworthy that in both treatment groups, the remaining calculus was generally found to be free of live bacteria. Thus, while neither method resulted in complete calculus removal, both methods were remarkably effective in bacterial debridement of subgingival root surfaces (Breininger et al., 1987).

More recently, 12 extracted mandibular incisors, each with similar levels of clinical root calculus were instrumented by either a manual curette or an ultrasonic tip until no visible calculus remained. Photomicrographs obtained via scanning electron microscopy were used to determine and compare levels of remaining calculus following each method of instrumentation. Assessment of the residual calculus showed no difference between the root surfaces treated by manual or ultrasonic instrumentation (Marda et al., 2012).

Thus, it seems reasonable to conclude that ultrasonic and manual instrumentation have equal capability to remove calculus. Neither method resulted in complete calculus removal. However, as reviewed in the first chapter and further detailed in the next section, both methods removed sufficient calculus during use to result in resolution of periodontal disease.

Biofilm removal

Early studies confirm the ability for both manual and ultrasonic instrumentation to have equivalent beneficial effects on the periodontal etiology (Thornton and Garnick, 1982; Oosterwaal et al., 1987; Renvert et al., 1990), with ultrasonic

Table 2.1 Microbial changes at 3 and 6 months after root debridement via manual (MI) and ultrasonic (USD) instrumentation

Species/Instrumentation method		Mean numbers ($\times 10^5$, mean $\pm$ SEM) of the four species tested		
		Baseline	3 months	6 months
Pg	MI	7.36 ± 2.29	2.63 ± 0.72[1]	1.39 ± 0.44[1]
	USD	5.45 ± 0.99	2.76 ± 0.69[1]	2.45 ± 0.59[1]
Aa	MI	1.51 ± 0.43	2.21 ± 0.53	0.99 ± 0.19
	USD	1.745 ± 0.69	1.94 ± 0.71	1.66 ± 0.49
Tf	MI	4.20 ± 1.57	0.75 ± 0.28	0.83 ± 0.24
	USD	3.06 ± 0.73	1.29 ± 0.49	2.44 ± 0.61[1]
Td	MI	3.03 ± 1.54	0.88 ± 0.23	0.74 ± 0.38
	USD	2.64 ± 0.073	1.05 ± 0.41	3.18 ± 1.21

Pg, *Porphyromonas gingivalis*; Aa, *Aggregatibacter actinomycetemcomitans*; Tf, *Tannerella forsythia*; Td, *Treponema denticola*.
[1] Statistically significant difference from baseline (Wilcoxon's Signed Ranks test, $p < 0.05$).
Source: Data from Ioannou et al., 2009.

instrumentation possibly offering an advantage in bacterial removal in furcation areas (Leon and Vogel, 1987).

Laboratory methods for bacterial identification have been refined considerably compared to the methods that were available at the time of these early studies. In a more recent study, DNA hybridization was employed to assess microbiological changes following manual and ultrasonic instrumentation (Iannou et al., 2009). Changes in levels of the so-called red complex pathogens that play a key role in periodontal disease development (Socransky et al., 1998) were assessed over a 6-month period. Teeth were treated either via manual instrumentation using a variety of curettes or by ultrasonic instrumentation using a piezoelectric device. In both cases, instrumentation continued until a "smooth, hard" surface was achieved as assessed clinically by using an explorer.

In alignment with the results of earlier studies, microbiological samples obtained at baseline and at 3 and 6 months demonstrate that manual and ultrasonic instrumentation are comparable in their ability to alter the periodontal bacteria (Table 2.1).

To optimize the mechanical disruption of biofilm, particularly at the microscopic level,

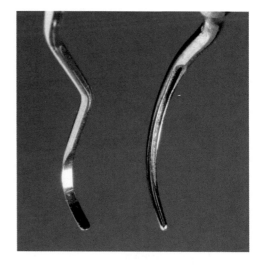

Figure 2.1 Comparison of the bladed, linear working end of a curette to the blunt, cylindrical active area of an ultrasonic tip

maximum contact between the tooth surface and the working end of the tip is required, regardless of the type of instrument used. It is here, relative to biofilm disruption, that the mechanisms of action and tip design inherent to ultrasonic instrumentation provide distinct advantages over manual instrumentation.

Manual instruments were designed with a bladed edge (Figure 2.1) primarily to cut calcified deposits and plane contaminated cementum from the tooth surface, with the resulting plaque removal being incidental. Using a bladed instrument at an appropriate force to remove the biofilm without cementum removal, while difficult in itself, requires constant effort to adequately adapt the straight cutting edge to the curvatures of the tooth and only results in biofilm interruption at the point of contact. To achieve maximum contact, the cutting edge of the instrument must be honed throughout the procedure. The integrity of the cutting edge is altered with contact between the blade and tooth/deposit/restoration surfaces. When altered, at the ultrastructural level, gaps where no contact is made between the edge and the root surface result, essentially leaving some portions of the root receiving only minimal debridement.

Conversely, the cylindrical shape of the blunt ultrasonic tip (Figure 2.1) is more conducive to biofilm removal than the linear cutting edge of a manual instrument, as it naturally conforms to the curvatures of the tooth surface (Chapter 4), and the biophysical forces of cavitation and microstreaming extend the interruption of biofilm beyond the point of direct tip contact (Chapter 3).

The advantages of ultrasonic instrumentation as described above are never more evident than during the debridement of furcations. There is general agreement among clinicians that effective instrumentation is considerably more difficult to achieve in areas of furcation involvement. It is of interest to note that studies in root morphology have shown that the measured entrance to furcation areas is often less than the blade width of curettes (Hou et al., 1994). This can severely limit the accessibility of furcations to thorough debridement with manual instrumentation.

In a study comparing manual and ultrasonic debridement of 33 molar furcations in 6 adult patients, ultrasonic and manual instrumentation were equally effective in reducing microbial counts (via dark field microscopy) in class I furcations. However, ultrasonic instrumentation was clearly superior in decreasing inflammation and motile forms of bacteria in class II and class III furcations (Leon and Vogel, 1987). Hence, ultrasonic devices may be the instruments of choice for debriding furcation and other areas with challenging root morphologies (Patterson et al., 1989; Oda and Ishikawa, 1989; Takacs et al., 1993).

In summary, although studies demonstrate that both manual and ultrasonic instrumentation sufficiently interrupt biofilm, the improved conformity afforded by the design of ultrasonic tips combined with the mechanisms of ultrasonic debridement (vibratory and biophysical) increases the likelihood that the biofilm will be disrupted below the threshold necessary to result in resolution of disease.

RESOLUTION OF DISEASE

The typical parameters that are assessed to determine the presence or progression of periodontal disease include probing depth, clinical attachment level (CAL), and inflammation (usually measured by BOP). The effect that ultrasonic or hand instrumentation has on these common parameters has been widely studied. While it is admittedly difficult to standardize all variables (e.g., operator skill level, time allotted per tooth or per arch, specific instrument type, type of deposits, morphology of involved roots), some generalizations can be made to determine the usefulness of the various debridement modalities. With the data demonstrating comparable efficacy of manual and ultrasonic instrumentation to remove root deposits in mind, it is reasonable to expect both methods of instrumentation to result in similar levels of clinical improvement.

Probing depth

A systematic review of 27 studies indicated that mean probing depth reductions following hand instrumentation ranged from 1.29 mm for pockets with moderate probing depth to 2.16 mm

Table 2.2a Mean changes in probing depth (PD) resulting from manual (MI) and ultrasonic (UI) instrumentation

Study	Method	Reduction in PD (mm)
Torfason et al., 1979	MI	1.70
	UI	1.72
Badersten et al., 1981	MI	1.0
	UI	1.2
Badersten et al., 1984	MI	1.4
	UI	1.2
Copulos et al., 1993	MI	0.72
	UI	0.75
Boretti et al., 1995	MI	1.83
	UI	1.82
Kocher et al., 2001	MI	0.77
	UI	1.10
Ioannou et al., 2009	MI	0.88
	UI	0.44

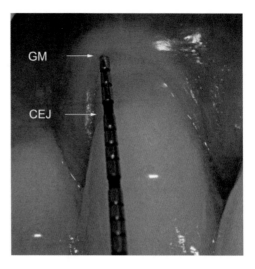

Figure 2.2 Probe indicates PD = 1 mm, with 4 mm of recession; thus, CAL = 5 mm. GM: gingival margin; CEJ: cementoenamel junction

for pockets with deep probing depths (Cobb, 1996). Studies that assessed probing depth reduction following the use of ultrasonic and sonic instruments yielded results almost identical to those achieved by manual instrumentation (Torfason et al., 1979; Badersten et al., 1981, 1984; Copulos et al., 1993; Boretti, 1995; Kocher, 2001, Ioannou et al., 2009) (Table 2.2a).

There is little doubt that a reduction in the pocket depth improves access to subgingival areas for the therapist and patient alike. Root surfaces adjacent to shallow pockets are more easily accessed by clinical instrumentation during debridement and by the patient during daily hygiene efforts. Therefore, reduction of probing depth is a laudable treatment goal as it reduces the likelihood of relapse. However, focusing the management of periodontal disease solely on pocket depth may not be sufficient.

Attachment level

Compared to probing depth, CAL is the more accurate indicator of the amount of periodontal tissue destruction that has taken place (Figure 2.2). Posttreatment, CAL allows the examiner to determine if a positive change in probing depth is due to a gain in periodontal attachment or simply due to recession of the soft tissues.

As with probing depth, gains in CAL are comparable between ultrasonic/sonic and manual debridement in the treatment of periodontitis (Badersten et al., 1981, 1984; Copulos et al., 1993; Boretti, 1995; Kocher, 2001; Ioannou, 2009) (Table 2.2b). Thus, both manual and ultrasonic instrumentation have the potential to not only reduce pocket depth but also to result in gains in clinical attachment.

Inflammation

Periodontal inflammation is initiated and perpetuated by the subgingival biofilm. It is the inflammatory response that causes the majority of the tissue breakdown, which results in the clinical signs and symptoms of periodontitis. Realizing that reduction of inflammation is now a goal of periodontal therapy, it seems prudent to assess the ability for manual and ultrasonic instrumentation to reduce inflammation as measured

Table 2.2b Mean changes in disease parameters resulting from manual (MI) and ultrasonic (UI) instrumentation

Study	Method	Reduction in PD (mm)	Gain in CAL (mm)	Reduction in % of sites with BOP
Torfason et al., 1979	MI	1.70		45%
	UI	1.72		45%
Badersten et al., 1981	MI	1.0	1.39 ± 0.44	64%
	UI	1.2	2.45 ± 0.59	63%
Badersten et al., 1984	MI	1.4	0.99 ± 0.19	51%
	UI	1.2	1.66 ± 0.49	52%
Copulos et al., 1993	MI	0.72	0.74 ± 0.38	
	UI	0.75	3.18 ± 1.21	
Boretti et al., 1995	MI	1.83	1.53	91%
	UI	1.82	1.14	91%
Kocher et al., 2001	MI	0.77	0.83 ± 0.24	42.7%
	UI	1.10	2.44 ± 0.61	56.9%
Ioannou et al., 2009	MI	0.88	0.50	
	UI	0.44	0.26	

by BOP. Similar to the other clinical markers of periodontal disease activity, both manual instrumentation and ultrasonic instrumentation have been shown to be comparable (Table 2.2b) in terms of posttreatment reductions in BOP (Torfason et al., 1979; Badersten et al., 1981, 1984; Boretti, 1995; Kocher, 2001).

CONSERVATION OF TOOTH STRUCTURE

At this point, we have established that manual and ultrasonic instrumentation are comparably effective at removing deposits and facilitating resolution of disease as measured by PD, CAL, and BOP. But, that is only part of the story. Remember, the goal of periodontal debridement is resolution of disease without excessive cementum removal. So, the next question to ask is, "which method is best suited to accomplish the objectives of periodontal therapy without over-instrumentation?"

As previously noted, manual instruments, the designs of which have not changed considerably over the years, were designed with a bladed edge with the intention of breaking calculus at the tooth–calculus interface and the removal (planing) of what was thought to be contaminated cementum. Inherent to the design of the instrument and the mechanism of deposit removal, the amount of root surface removed during debridement with a bladed instrument can be significant.

Root surface damage

Studies that assess root damage are difficult to compare owing to variations in measurement techniques, stroke length, instrument pressure, time used, instrument tip integrity (e.g., sharpness), and so on (Proceedings of the 1996 World Workshop). Despite these limitations, some trends have become evident.

Studies have consistently shown that root planing with manual instruments removes more cementum than when using ultrasonic instruments, and can result in removal of far more than the maximum of 50 μm of cementum per year suggested by Flemmig et al. (1998a,b). For example, in a study assessing four different

Treatment	Application Force (p)	Mean loss of substance (μm) after 12 strokes	Loss of substance (μm) per working stroke
Ultrasonic scaler	100	11.6 (8.0 – 15.1)	1.0
Air scaler	100	93.5 (84.2 – 102.7)	7.8
Fine curette	500	108.9 (101.8 – 116.0)	9.1
Diamond bur	100	118.7 (114.1 – 123.4)	9.9

Figure 2.3 Loss of root substance resulting from various instruments. Data compiled from information found in Ritz et al., 1991

methods of debridement (Figure 2.3), the mean cementum removal when using a manual instrument was 108.9 μm, compared to 11.6 μm when using an ultrasonic instrument, following just 12 working strokes applied with clinically appropriate force at 360 sites on 90 extracted mandibular incisors (Ritz et al., 1991).

In another study of 48 extracted teeth, after 30 instrument strokes, 33.2 μm of root structure was removed by hand instruments, compared to 21.6 μm when using an ultrasonic insert (Vastardis et al., 2005). When using a manual instrument applied with a force of 3 N (which is less than the clinical norm), the mean cumulative root substance loss was 148.7 μm after 40 strokes, and this increased to 343.3 μm (i.e., more than one-third of a millimeter) after 40 strokes at forces of 8.5 N (Zappa et al., 1991). It is unclear if the degree of root alterations varies among the myriad of differing manual scaling instruments.

Furthermore, if root planing is undertaken on several occasions, there is a cumulative removal of cementum and eventually, cementum may be completely removed from areas of the root surface (Figure 2.4).

The obvious major disadvantage of manual instrumentation is that tooth substance (i.e., cementum) is physically removed, and the main consequence of this is dentin sensitivity.

Although it has been reported that root planing creates a smear layer that reduces the permeability of the underlying dentin (Fogel and Pashley, 1993), this smear layer is acid labile,

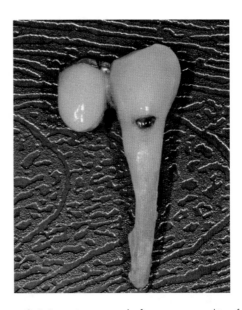

Figure 2.4 Extensive removal of cementum resulting from multiple courses of root planing. Image courtesy of Dr. Ian Dunn, Liverpool, UK

and therefore root planing may ultimately cause increased dentin permeability resulting in dentin sensitivity, bacterial invasion of dentinal tubules, and pulpal irritation.

A significant increase in root surface roughness and/or loss resulting from sonic scalers compared to ultrasonic scalers has been demonstrated (Ritz et al., 1991; Jotkasthira et al., 1992; Jacobson et al., 1994; Schmidlin et al., 2001). This increase in root surface alteration is attributed to the higher degree of force resulting from longer strokes of oscillation (higher displacement amplitude), and is likely exacerbated by the wider-diameter tips commonly used with sonic scalers. While the sonic scaler has demonstrated efficacy comparable to ultrasonic and hand instruments in calculus removal (Lie and Leknes, 1985; Jotkasthira et al., 1992) and resolution of the clinical signs of periodontal disease (Loos et al., 1987, 1989; Laurell and Pettersson, 1988; Christgau et al., 2006), the resulting degree of root surface damage is unacceptable and contraindicates the use of the sonic scaler for root surface debridement, limiting its clinical application to coronal calculus removal.

Debridement of dental implants

As with natural teeth, bacterial accumulations on dental implant surfaces can induce inflammatory changes in the supporting tissues that may lead to the loss of supporting bone and ultimately implant loss (Figure 2.5) (Esposito et al., 2010). Because peri-implant pathology is associated with biofilm formation, the elimination of biofilm is essential in the management and control of peri-implant infections. Long-term

maintenance care, including regular debridement of implant surfaces, is essential to reduce the risk of peri-implant pathology (Atieh et al., 2012). Similarly to root surfaces, bacterial colonization on implant surfaces is influenced, in part, by surface roughness. (Rimondini et al., 1997). Damage to implant surfaces secondary to debridement can adversely affect the biocompatibility of the implant (Fox et al., 1990). While there are differences between natural teeth and dental implants in terms of the architecture at the implant–soft tissue interface (Donley and Gillette, 1991), the prerequisites for debridement are similar to those for the natural dentition: effective and efficient removal of as much clinical and microscopic etiology as possible in a manner that retains the integrity of the implant surface (Renvert et al., 2009).

Perhaps it would be most appropriate to substitute the commonly used clinical term, "implant maintenance" with the more descriptive term, "implant surface maintenance." Because of the different components involved in implant prosthetics, the surfaces in need of debridement may include smooth or rough implant titanium surfaces; abutments composed of titanium or other

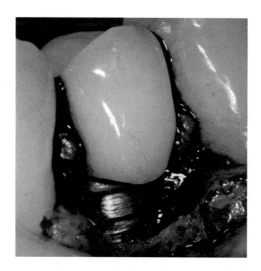

Figure 2.5 Bone deterioration secondary to peri-implantitis

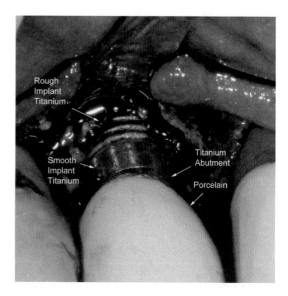

Figure 2.6 Various materials and textures of different components of an implant

materials; and crown restorations fabricated out of porcelain, metal, or other restorative materials Figure 2.6). The effect of ultrasonic instrumentation on other restorative materials that may be encountered during maintenance of implants or natural teeth is addressed in Chapter 5.

Effect of instrumentation

Comparisons between the debridement capabilities of ultrasonic and manual instrumentation methods may be of secondary interest because studies consistently find that both metal curettes and metal ultrasonic tips result in an unacceptable level of surface damage to the titanium surface of the implant or implant abutment. (Louropoulou et al., 2013). It is generally agreed that metal curettes and ultrasonic tips should not be used routinely to maintain either smooth or rough titanium surfaces. Many implant surfaces are purposely rough by design to promote osseointegration. In cases of peri-implantitis, the rough implant threads can become exposed to oral microorganisms and bacterial colonization of the titanium surface can occur, leading to the loss of osseointegration. In addition to decontamination of the exposed surface, treatment also includes smoothing the exposed rough titanium in an effort to make it less plaque-retentive. Metal instruments have been shown to be effective in cases requiring smoothing of an exposed rough titanium surface (Louropoulou et al., 2012).

Alternatives to ultrasonic metal tips are being explored to determine if they can be used to achieve adequate debridement without any surface damage (Unursaikhan, 2012; Ruhling et al., 1994; Kawashima et al., 2007). In recent years, ultrasonic and sonic tips composed of carbon fiber or with disposable plastic covers have been developed specifically for the debridement of implant surfaces (Figure 2.7). Studies have demonstrated that these nonmetal tips do not alter smooth titanium surfaces (Sato et al., 2004; Kawashima et al., 2007; Mann et al., 2012), but can cause significant surface disruption of

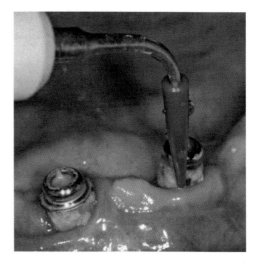

Figure 2.7 Example of a plastic-covered implant-specific ultrasonic tip

both plasma and hydroxyapatite coated surfaces (Thomson-Neal et al., 1989; Augthun et al., 1998; Bailey et al., 1998; Ramaglia et al., 2006). While it is tempting to assume that the debridement efficacy of a plastic-covered tip parallels that of a traditional ultrasonic tip, the potential of an attached plastic cover to affect the oscillatory movement of the tip has to be considered.

Mann et al. (2012) assessed the oscillation patterns and effect on titanium implant surfaces of both a traditional ultrasonic tip and an implant-specific insert with a disposable plastic tip. Using a scanning laser vibrometry, the oscillation patterns of the traditional and plastic covered tips were found to be similar. Inadequate attachment of the plastic covering to the insert tip tended to reduce the vibration amplitude. The effect of this reduced mechanical action on the performance of the tip has not been measured. Likewise, the production of cavitation and microstreaming forces by nonmetal ultrasonic tips has not been assessed.

The plastic cover minimized any damage to the implant surface as assessed by laser profilometry. However, SEM analysis suggested that the plastic-covered tips did result in some degree of implant surface alteration. While no volume of material was removed from the titanium surface, the tips exhibited a "polishing" effect. At higher power, the plastic cover tended to melt and portions of this melted plastic adhered to the implant surface. The authors cautioned that using the plastic-covered tip against the edges of roughened titanium (e.g., exposed implant threads) may result in shredding of the plastic with even greater deposits left behind. Any clinical ramifications of this residual plastic have not yet been investigated.

Protective plastic covers by design tend to be bulky and difficult to introduce into the subgingival environment adjacent to implant surfaces. While it certainly seems reasonable to harness the benefits of ultrasonic debridement when treating implant surfaces, current designs may need to be modified to reduce any dampening of the oscillatory effect, permit better access, and allow effective debridement without producing any residual debris.

OTHER ADVANTAGES OF ULTRASONIC INSTRUMENTATION

Efficiency

An additional potential benefit of using ultrasonic instrumentation is reduced treatment time compared to manual instrumentation. As reviewed earlier in this chapter and in Chapter 1, it is not possible to determine the success of instrumentation at the time the instrumentation is completed. Instrumentation is performed until any clinically detectable deposits and as much microscopic etiology as possible are removed. The success of the procedure is determined only by assessing the soft tissue response to therapy after an adequate period of healing. Factors that affect the amount of time involved in the actual instrumentation include root morphology, the characteristics of any root deposit, the type of instrument being used, and the skill of the clinician. Thus, it is not possible to determine an actual time necessary to "scale or root plane"

a tooth. However, the results from studies in which treatment time/method was assessed (and in which the eventual response to therapy was deemed as clinically successful), can provide insight into the difference between methods in treatment time necessary to obtain a clinically acceptable result. Several studies have shown that debridement time spent per tooth may be reduced when ultrasonics are utilized compared to manual instrumentation (Copulos et al., 1993; Boretti et al., 1995; Dahiyaespoist and Kamal, 2012).

OTHER METHODS OF DEBRIDEMENT

Laser

The ability for laser-generated energy to disrupt biofilm continues to be a popular topic of discussion in periodontics. Laser is an acronym, which stands for light amplification by stimulated emission of radiation. A laser is a device that converts electrical or chemical energy into an emitted beam of light energy. Typically, lasers are named according to the active elements that are induced to create the energy beam. The most common laser wavelengths that have been suggested to be of benefit during periodontal therapy include diode, CO_2, ND:YAG, ER:YAG, and Er,Cr:YSGG (Figure 2.8).

When laser energy is directed at biologic tissue, the laser energy is largely absorbed by the target tissue. The absorbed light energy is converted to heat which can result in warming

Type of laser	Wavelength in nanometers (nm)
Diode	809–980
Nd:YAG	1064
Er,Cr:YSGG	2780
Er:YAG	2940
CO2	10,600

Figure 2.8 Laser wavelengths with periodontal application

of the tissue, coagulation, or excision of tissue through vaporization. The generated heat also has the potential to provide a bactericidal effect. The degree of tissue absorption depends in part on variable laser characteristics including wavelength of the emitted light, power (watts), waveform, pulse duration, energy/pulse, energy density, duration of exposure, peak power of pulse, and angulation of the energy delivery tip to the target surface. Periodontal target tissue characteristics will also determine the effect that the laser energy will have on the tissue as each wavelength of laser energy is absorbed to a greater or lesser degree in water, pigment, or hydroxyapatite. In general, shorter wavelength lasers (diode and Nd:Yag) have a higher affinity for pigmented tissues and a low absorption coefficient in water, which makes them more likely to penetrate deeper into soft tissues. Other factors that likely affect what happens when laser energy is directed at periodontal tissues include the degree of tissue inflammation and vascularity, and the availability of progenitor cells to participate in the healing process (Cobb, 2006).

Laser curettage

Because specific laser wavelengths affect periodontal tissues differently, various laser types have been suggested as being beneficial in the effort to affect biofilm or remove calculus. Specific laser energy can be used to target specific periodontal tissues such as lining epithelium. However, as established in Chapter 1, "gingival curettage" via any methods has repeatedly been shown to have no significant therapeutic effect. Not surprisingly, a review of the available evidence does not support the use of laser-induced removal of the epithelial pocket lining during periodontal debridement (Cobb et al., 2010; Karlsson et al., 2008).

Laser debridement

In terms of periodontal debridement, the question as to whether the use of laser for debridement provides any advantages when used either as a stand-alone therapy or as an adjunct to ultrasonic debridement is far from settled. Lasers would be most useful as a method of periodontal debridement if laser energy could be harnessed to affect bacteria and/or root deposits without any collateral tissue damage. Many early studies concerning the bactericidal potential of various laser energies were done *in vitro* and may not correlate to the clinical development of a periodontal biofilm. Laboratory replication of the complex structure of a periodontal biofilm is challenging. Comparisons of the debridement potential of various lasers are also difficult as studies vary in how the laser energy is delivered (e.g., sweeping motion or static delivery into the pocket), the power or energy density being utilized, whether the energy is delivered in a single or multiple pulse, and the angle of delivery of irradiation relative to the root surface (Cobb, 2006). Current evidence show lasers, as a group, to be unpredictable and inconsistent in their ability to reduce subgingival microbial loads beyond that achieved by SRP alone (Karlsson et al., 2008; Schwarz et al., 2008; Cobb et al., 2010).

Calculus removal with laser

If using laser energy for removal of calcified root deposits, the wavelength of the selected laser should effectively remove calculus while avoiding any thermal damage to adjacent pulp or root tissues and any unnecessary removal of sound root structure. Of the available lasers, the Er:YAG laser would seem to be the best choice due to its wavelength characteristics that result in minimal penetration into mineralized tissue. While evidence suggests that removal of calcified deposits via laser energy is possible (Schwarz et al., 2008), distinguishing between cementum and clinically detectable calculus or even microscopic calculus (especially during nonsurgical therapy) is at best, challenging. Certainly, further study will be necessary to determine if laser energy can be used for hard deposit removal

Table 2.3 Comparison of ultrasonic and manual instrumentation in meeting the objectives of periodontal debridement

Objective	Method of Greater Efficacy	Comments
Disruption and removal of subgingival biofilm	**Ultrasonic**	*Although both methods are equal in capability, ultrasonic debridement is preferred because the design of the tip permits improved access and the biophysical mechanisms increase the predictability of biofilm disruption*
Conservation of tooth structure	**Ultrasonic**	*When used properly, ultrasonic instrumentation results in significantly less root surface removal during instrumentation*
Removal of calculus	**Equal**	*Although both methods are equally capable of removing calculus, ultrasonic instrumentation is preferred because the calculus is more likely to be removed without excessive alteration of the root surface*
Resolution of inflammation	**Equal**	*While both methods are equally capable of facilitating resolution of the inflammation, resolution without concurrent root surface damage is more difficult to achieve with manual instrumentation*
Efficiency	**Ultrasonic**	*In studies, less time was necessary to achieve the desired clinical outcome when using ultrasonic instrumentation as compared to manual instrumentation*

without resulting in concomitant damage to the adjacent tissues. Further complicating the selection of the ideal laser parameters for efficacious calculus removal is the differential susceptibility to damage of calculus, cementum, and dentin (even within the same specimen) due to variability in the color, thickness, composition, texture, and water content of the specimen (Radvar et al., 1995; Cobb, 2006).

Despite an ever-increasing inclusion of lasers into clinical periodontal protocols, deriving evidence-based conclusions is still not possible. The quality and quantity of evidence necessary in the evidence-based approach (Forrest and Overman, 2013) simply does not yet exist. While laser energy has the potential to play a role in periodontal therapy, it is not yet possible to recommend a predictable protocol utilizing a controlled delivery of a specific laser wavelength

to selectively ablate calculus or disrupt biofilm. In their systematic review of the evidence investigating laser use in periodontal therapy, Cobb et al. (2010) asked a salient question; "Is the current use of dental lasers for the treatment of periodontitis based on peer-reviewed evidence obtained under controlled conditions or word of mouth, unconfirmed evidence?" At the time of publication of this text, the question remains unanswered.

Summary

At the time of this publication, the profession has yet to complete the shift from manual to ultrasonic instrumentation as the primary method of debridement, seeming to favor instead a combined approach that uses both ultrasonic and manual instruments. The reasons for the combined approach likely being an unwillingness to let go of long-held misperceptions about the superiority of manual instrumentation combined with the common practice of utilizing only one ultrasonic tip design ("universal"), which requires supplemental manual instrumentation because of the inability of the universal tip design to access all root surfaces. A lack of training and/or instructional resources specific to ultrasonic instrumentation may also play a role. The benefits of a combined approach in terms of periodontal outcomes have not been widely studied. Despite the lack of evidence, advocacy for the combined approach perpetuates in the profession.

Biofilm disruption can be accomplished by manual instrumentation, laser generated energy, and ultrasonic instrumentation. However, a solid understanding of the evidence base demonstrating the effectiveness and advantages of ultrasonic instrumentation in meeting the objectives of periodontal debridement (Table 2.3) can only lead to the acceptance of ultrasonic technology as the primary method of nonsurgical periodontal debridement.

REFERENCES

American Dental Association Center for Evidence-Based Dentistry. Available at: "www.http://ebd.ada.org/About.aspx". Accessed 14 July 2013.

Apatzidou DA, Kinane DF. Nonsurgical mechanical treatment strategies for periodontal disease. *Dent Clin North Am* 2010; 54: 1–12.

Atieh MA, Alsabeeha NH, Faggion CM Jr, Duncan WJ. The frequency of peri-implant diseases: a systematic review and meta-analysis. *J Periodontol* 2013; 84: 1586–98.

Augthun M, Tinschert J, Huber A. In vitro studies on the effect of cleaning methods on different implant surfaces. *J Periodontol* 1998; 69: 857–64.

Bader J, Ismail A. ADA Council on Scientific Affairs; Division of Science; Journal of the American Dental Association. Survey of systematic reviews in dentistry. *J Am Dent Assoc.* 2004; 135: 464–73.

Badersten A, Nilveus R., Egelberg J. Effect of nonsurgical periodontal therapy. I. Moderately advanced periodontitis. *J Clin Periodontol* 1981; 8: 57–72.

Badersten A, Nilveus, R., Egelberg J. Effect of non-surgical periodontal therapy. II. Severely advanced periodontitis. *J Clin Periodontol* 1984; 11: 63–76.

Bailey GM, Gardner JS, Day MH, Kovanda BJ. Implant surface alterations from a nonmetallic ultrasonic tip. *J West Soc Periodontol Periodontal Abstr* 1998; 46: 69–73.

Benfenati MP, Montesani MT, Benfenati SP, Nathanson D. Scanning electron microscope: an SEM study of periodontally instrumented root surfaces, comparing sharp, dull, and damaged curettes and ultrasonic instruments. *Int J Periodontics Restorative Dent* 1987; 7: 50–67.

Bergenholtz G, Lindhe J. Effect of experimental induced marginal periodontitis and periodontal scaling on the dental pulp. *J Clin Periodontal.* 1979; 5: 59–73.

Boretti G, Zappa U, Graf H, Case D, et al., Short-term effects of phase I therapy on crevicular cell populations. *J Periodontol* 1995; 66: 235–40.

Breininger DR, O'Leary TJ, Blumenshine RV. Comparative effectiveness of ultrasonic and hand scaling for the removal of subgingival plaque and calculus. *J Periodontol* 1987; 58: 9–18.

Chapple IL, Walmsley AD, Saxby MS, Moscrop H. Effect of instrument power setting during ultrasonic scaling upon treatment outcome. *J Periodontol* 1995; 66: 756–60.

Christgau M, Männer T, Beuer S, Hiller KA, Schmalz G. Periodontal healing after non-surgical therapy with a modified sonic scaler: a controlled clinical trial. *J Clin Periodontol* 2006; 33: 749–58.

Cobb CM. Non-surgical pocket therapy: Mechanical. *Ann Periodontol* 1996; 61: 443–90.

Cobb CM. Lasers in periodontics: a review of the literature. *J Periodontol* 2006; 77: 545–64.

Cobb CM, Low SB, Coluzzi DJ. Lasers and the treatment of chronic periodontitis. *Dent Clin N Am* 2010; 54: 35–53.

Copulos TA, Low SB, Walker CB, Trebilcock YY, Hefti AF. Comparative analysis between a modified ultrasonic tip and hand instruments on clinical parameters of periodontal disease. *J Periodontol* 1993; 64: 694–700.

Dahiya P, Kamal R. Ultra-morphology of root surface subsequent to periodontal instrumentation: A scanning electron microscope study. *J Indian Soc Periodontol* 2012; 16: 96–100.

Donley TG, Gillette WB. Titanium endosseous implant-soft tissue interface: a literature review. *J Periodontol* 1991; 62: 153–60.

Drisko CH. Dentine hypersensitivity – dental hygiene and periodontal considerations. *Int Dent J* 2002; 52: 385–93.

Dragoo MR. A clinical evaluation of hand and ultrasonic instruments on subgingival debridement. 1. With unmodified and modified ultrasonic inserts. *Int J Periodontics Restorative Dent.* 1992; 12: 310–23.

Esposito M, Grusovin MG, Polyzos IP, Felice P, Worthington HV. Interventions for replacing missing teeth: dental implants in fresh extraction sockets (immediate, immediate-delayed and delayed implants). *Cochrane Database Syst Rev.* 2010 Sep 8; (9). (Published online).

Flemmig TF, Petersilka GJ, Mehl A, Hickel R, Klaiber B. The effect of working parameters on root substance removal using a piezoelectric ultrasonic scaler in vitro. *J Clin Periodontol* 1998a; 25: 158–63.

Flemmig TF, Petersilka GJ, Mehl A, Hickel R, Klaiber B. Working parameters of a magnetostrictive ultrasonic scaler influencing root substance removal in vitro. *J Periodontol* 1998b; 69: 547–53.

Fogel HM, Pashley DH. Effect of periodontal root planing on dentin permeability. *J Clin Periodontol* 1993; 20: 673–7.

Forrest JL, Overman P. Keeping current: A commitment to patient care excellence through evidence based practice. *J Dent Hyg* 2013, 87: 33–40.

Fox SC, Moriarty JD, Kusy RP. The effects of scaling a titanium implant surface with metal and plastic instruments: an in vitro study. *J Periodontol* 1990: 485–90.

Gantes BG, Nilveus R The effect of different hygiene instruments on titanium surfaces: SEM observations. *Int J Periodontics Restorative Dent* 1991; 11: 225–39.

Hallmon WW, Rees TD. Local anti-infective therapy: mechanical and physical approaches. A systematic review. *Ann Periodontol* 2003; 8: 99–114.

Hunter RK, O'Leary TJ, Kafrawy AH. The effectiveness of hand versus ultrasonic instrumentation in open flap root planing. *J Periodontol* 1984; 55: 697–703.

Hou GL, Chen SF, Wu YM, Tsai CC. The topography of the furcation entrance in Chinese molars. Furcation entrance dimensions. *J Clin Periodontol* 1994; 21: 451–6.

Ioannou I, Dimitriadis N, Papadimitriou K, Sakellari D, Vouros I, Konstantinidis A. Hand instrumentation versus ultrasonic debridement in the treatment of chronic periodontitis. a randomized clinical and microbiological trial. *J Clin Periodontol* 2009; 36: 132–41.

Jacobson L, Blomlöf J, Lindskog S. Root surface texture after different scaling modalities. *Scand J Dent Res* 1994; 102: 156–60.

Jotikasthira NE, Lie T, Leknes KN. Comparative in vitro studies of sonic, ultrasonic and reciprocating scaling instruments. *J Clin Periodontol* 1992; 19: 560–9.

Karlsson MR, Lofgren CD, Jansson HM. The effect of laser therapy as an adjunct to non-surgical periodontal treatment in subjects with chronic periodontitis: a systematic review. *J Periodontol* 2008; 79: 2021–8.

Kawashima H, Sato S, Kishida M, Yagi H, Matsumoto K, Ito K. Treatment of titanium dental implants with three piezoelectric ultrasonic scalers: an in vivo study. *J Periodontol* 2007, 78: 1689–94.

Kepic TJ, O'Leary TJ, Kafrawy AH. Total calculus removal: an attainable objective? *J Periodontol* 1990; 61: 16–20.

Kocher T, Konig J, Hansen P, Ruhling A Subgingival polishing compared with scaling with steel curettes: a clinical pilot study. *J Clin Periodontol* 2001: 8; 194–9.

Laurell L, Pettersson B. Periodontal healing after treatment with either the Titan-S sonic scaler or hand instruments. *Swed Dent J* 1988; 12: 187–92.

Leon LE, Vogel RI. A comparison of the effectiveness of hand scaling and ultrasonic debridement in furcations as evaluated by differential dark-field microscopy. *J Periodontol* 1987; 58: 86–94.

Lie T, Leknes KN. Evaluation of the effect on root surfaces of air turbine scalers and ultrasonic instrumentation. *J Periodontol* 1985; 56: 522–31.

Loos B, Kiger R, Egelberg J. An evaluation of basic periodontal therapy using sonic and ultrasonic scalers. *J Clin Periodontol* 1987; 14: 29–33.

Loos B, Nylund K, Claffey N, et al., Clinical effects of root debridement in molar and non-molar teeth. A 2- year follow up. *J Clin Periodontol* 1989; 16: 498–504.

Louropoulou A, Slot DE, Van der Weijden FA. Titanium surface alterations following the use of different mechanical instruments: a systematic review. *Clin Oral Implants Res* 2012; 23: 643–58.

Louropoulou A, Slot DE, Van der Weijden F. The effects of mechanical instruments on contaminated titanium dental implant surfaces: a systematic review. *Clin Oral Implants Res.* 2013; Jul 8. [Epub ahead of print]

Mann M, Parmar D, Walmsley AD, Lea SC. Effect of plastic-covered ultrasonic scalers on titanium implant surfaces. *Clin Oral Implants Res* 2012; 231: 76–82.

Marda P, Prakash S, Devaraj C G, Vastardis S. A comparison of root surface instrumentation using manual, ultrasonic and rotary instruments: An in vitro study using scanning electron microscopy. *Indian J Dent Res* 2012; 23: 164–70.

Oda S, Ishikawa I. In vitro effectiveness of a newly-designed ultrasonic scaler tip for furcation areas. *J Periodontol* 1989; 60: 634–9.

Oosterwaal PJ, Matee MI, Mikx FH, van 't Hof MA, Renggli HH. The effect of subgingival debridement with hand and ultrasonic instruments on the subgingival microflora. *J Clin Periodontol.* 1987; 14: 528–33.

Patterson M, Eick JD, Eberhart AB, Gross K, Killoy WJ. The effectiveness of two sonic and two ultrasonic scaler tips in furcations. *J Periodontol* 1989; 60: 325–9.

Proceedings of the 1996 World Workshop in Periodontics. Lansdowne, Virginia, 13–17 July 1996. *Ann Periodontol* 1996 Nov; 1: 1–947.

Radvar M, Creanor SL, Gilmour WH, Payne AP, McGadey J, Foye RH, Whitters CJ, Kinane DF. An evaluation of the effects of an Nd:YAG laser on subgingival calculus, dentine and cementum. An in vitro study. *J Clin Periodontol* 1995; 22: 71–7.

Ramaglia L, di Lauro AE, Morgese F, Squillace A. Profilometric and standard error of the mean analysis of rough implant surfaces treated with different instrumentations. *Implant Dent* 2006; 15: 77–82.

Renvert S, Wikström M, Dahlén G, Slots J, Egelberg J. Effect of root debridement on the elimination of Actinobacillus actinomycetemcomitans and Bacteroides gingivalis from periodontal pockets. *J Clin Periodontol* 1990; 17: 345–50.

Rimondini L, Farè S, Brambilla E, Felloni A, Consonni C, Brossa F, Carrassi A. The effect of surface roughness on early in vivo plaque colonization on titanium. *J Periodontol* 1997; 68: 556–62.

Ritz L, Hefti AF, Rateitschak KH. An in vitro investigation on the loss of root substance in scaling with various instruments. *J Clin Periodontol* 1991; 18: 643–7.

Rosen PS Research, Science and Therapy Committee of the American Academy of Periodontology. Treatment of plaque-induced gingivitis, chronic periodontitis, and other clinical conditions. *J Periodontol* 2001; 72: 1790–1800.

Ruhling A, Kocher T, Kreusch J, Plagmann HC Treatment of subgingival implant surfaces with Teflon-coated sonic and ultrasonic scaler tips and various implant curettes. An in vitro study. *Clin Oral Implan Res* 1994; 5: 19–29.

Sato S, Kishida M, Ito K. The comparative effect of ultrasonic scalers on titanium surfaces: an in vitro study. *J Periodontol* 2004; 75: 1269–73.

Schwarz F, Aoki A, Becker J, Sculean A. Laser application in non-surgical periodontal therapy: a systematic review. *J Clin Periodontol* 2008; 35: 29–44.

Sbordone L, Ramaglia L, Guletta E, et al., Recolonization of the subgingival microflora after scaling and root planing in human periodontitis. *J Periodontol* 1990; 61: 579–84.

Schmage P, Thielemann J, Nergiz I, Scorziello T.M., Pfeiffer P. Effects of 10 cleaning instruments on four different implant surfaces. *Int J Oral Maxillofac Implant* 2012; 27: 308–17.

Schmidlin PR, Beuchat M, Busslinger A, Lehmann B, Lutz F. Tooth substance loss resulting from mechanical, sonic and ultrasonic root instrumentation assessed by liquid scintillation. *J Clin Periodontol* 2001; 28: 1058–66.

Socransky SS, Haffajee AD, Cugini MA, Smith C, Kent RL. Microbial complexes in subgingival plaque. *J Clin Periodontol* 1998; 25: 134–44.

Takacs VJ, Lie T, Perala DG, Adams DF. Efficacy of 5 machining instruments in scaling of molar furcations. *J Periodontol* 1993; 64: 228–36.

Thomson-Neal D, Evans GH, Meffert RM. Effects of various prophylactic treatments on titanium, sapphire, and hydroxyapatite-coated implants: an SEM study. *Int J Periodontics Restorative Dent* 1989; 9: 300–11.

Thornton S, Garnick J. Comparison of ultrasonic to hand instruments in the removal of subgingival plaque. *J Periodontol* 1982; 53: 35–7.

Torfason T, Kiger R, Selvig K, Egelberg J. Clinical improvement of gingival conditions following ultrasonic versus hand instrumentation of periodontal pockets. *J Clin Periodontol* 1979; 6: 165–76.

Tunkel J, Heinecke A, Flemmig TF. A systematic review of efficacy of machine-driven and manual subgingival debridement in the treatment of chronic periodontitis. *J Clin Periodontol* 2002; 29: 72–81.

Unursaikhan O, Lee JS, Cha JK, Park JC, Jung UW, Kim CS, Cho KS, Choi SH. Comparative evaluation of roughness of titanium surfaces treated by different hygiene instruments. *Periodontal Implant Sci* 2012; 42: 88–94.

Vastardis S, Yukna RA, Rice DA, Mercante D. Root surface removal and resultant surface texture with diamond-coated ultrasonic inserts: an in vitro and SEM study. *J Clin Periodontol* 2005; 32: 467–73.

Zappa U, Smith B, Simona C, Graf H, Case D, Kim W. Root substance removal by scaling and root planing. *J Periodontol* 1991; 62: 750–4.

COMPARISON OF PERIODONTAL DEBRIDEMENT INSTRUMENTATION MODALITIES

SECTION II

ULTRASONIC TECHNOLOGY

Chapter 3

What is ultrasonic instrumentation?

CHAPTER OBJECTIVES

On completion of this chapter, the student will be able to:

1. Differentiate between magnetostrictive and piezoelectric ultrasonic transduction.

2. Define the mechanisms of action by which ultrasonic instruments remove deposits from the tooth surface.

3. Explain the relationship of key operational variables to the acoustic power produced by the ultrasonic scaling unit.

4. Adjust the operational variables as necessary in order to operate the ultrasonic scaling unit at a level of acoustic power appropriate for the treatment objective.

As presented in Chapter 1, the objective of periodontal debridement is to reduce periodontal pathogens and promote periodontal health by disrupting and removing deposits, ranging from biofilm to calculus, without over-instrumentation of the root surface. Hand scaling instruments (sickles, curettes, files, hoes, and chisels) remove/disrupt the deposits by manually stroking a bladed cutting edge across the tooth surface to mechanically break the bond between the deposit and the tooth (Lea and Walmsley, 2009). Ultrasonic scaling instruments *oscillate* (move forward and backward) a typically blunt metal tip at a high-frequency producing mechanical vibratory, cavitational and acoustic microstreaming forces that remove/disrupt the deposits. (Walmsley et al., 1984; Khambay and Walmsley, 1999).

Sound is a form of energy produced by vibrations. Humans can hear sound at frequencies up to 20,000 Hz or 20 kHz. The term *ultrasonic* applies to sound (or *acoustic*) energy having a frequency greater than 20 kHz, above the range audible to the human ear (Walmsley, 1989). Ultrasound is used in many different fields, typically to penetrate a medium and measure the reflection signature (e.g., sonography used in obstetrics) or to supply focused energy (e.g., ultrasonic cleaning of jewelry) (Figure 3.1).

Ultrasonic dental instruments convert electrical current into high-frequency (25–30 kHz) mechanical vibrations (Lea and Walmsley, 2009). The conversion is attained by either a magnetostrictive or piezoelectric *transducer*.

Ultrasonic Periodontal Debridement: Theory and Technique, First Edition. Marie D. George, Timothy G. Donley and Philip M. Preshaw.
© 2014 John Wiley & Sons, Inc. Published 2014 by John Wiley & Sons, Inc.

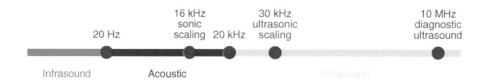

Figure 3.1 Range of sound frequencies. Frequencies >20 kHz are ultrasonic

ULTRASONIC TRANSDUCTION

Magnetostriction

Magnetostriction is defined as the changing of a material's physical dimensions in response to changing its magnetization. In other words, a magnetostrictive material will change shape when it is subjected to a magnetic field (Laird and Walmsley, 1991). Examples of magnetostrictive materials are iron, nickel, nickel alloys, and cobalt.

In ultrasonic dental devices, magnetostriction is attained by applying an alternating electromagnetic field to a stack of nickel strips. In response to the magnetization, the nickel stack elongates, then contracts along its length (i.e., changes

dimensions) producing longitudinal vibrations (Oda et al., 2004) (Figure 3.2). These vibrations travel from the stack through a connecting body to a tip, resulting in high-frequency oscillation of the tip (Figure 3.3).

The electromagnetic energy produced by magnetostrictive scaling units has been a topic of controversy with regard to any potential interaction with cardiac pacemakers. This issue is fully addressed in Chapter 5.

The components characteristic of magnetostrictive scaling units are listed in Table 3.1 and illustrated by Figures 3.4–3.8.

Piezoelectricity

Crystalline structures, such as quartz and certain ceramics, which undergo dimensional changes

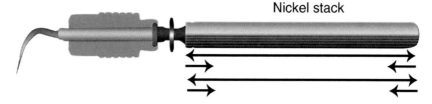

Figure 3.2 Diagram of a magnetostrictive insert. Application of an electromagnetic field to the stack of nickel strips results in magnetostriction – elongation then contraction – of the nickel stack along its length, producing longitudinal vibrations

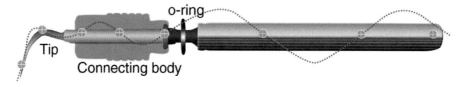

Figure 3.3 Longitudinal vibrations travel from the nickel stack through a connecting body to the tip of the insert. The crosshairs denote points of no vibration or movement, referred to as *nodal points* or *antinodes*

Table 3.1 Components of magnetostrictive ultrasonic units

Component	Description

Insert

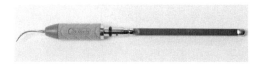

Composed of a *stack* of thin nickel strips soldered together at the ends and attached by a *connecting body* to a *tip*

Figure 3.4 A magnetostrictive insert

Handpiece

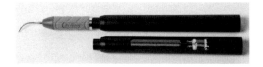

Holds the insert to surround the nickel stack in a spiral of copper wire which generates a magnetic field upon application of electrical current, resulting in magnetostriction of the stack

Figure 3.5 The handpiece of a magnetostrictive unit contains a spiral of copper wire (visible in the lower, cut-out handpiece), which surrounds the stack once the insert is seated in the handpiece

Base unit

Houses controls which regulate power level and water flow; provides connection between foot switch and handpiece

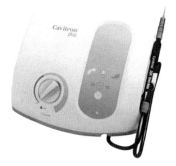

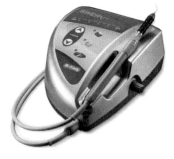

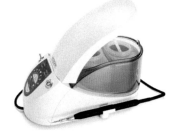

Figure 3.8 Integra™ magnetostrictive scaler (Image courtesy of Parkell, Inc).

Figure 3.6 Cavitron® plus magnetostrictive scaler (Image courtesy of Dentsply Professional)

Figure 3.7 SWERV® magnetostrictive scaler (Image courtesy of Hu-Friedy Mfg Co., LLC, Chicago IL, USA)

Foot switch

When engaged, sends electrical current through base unit to the handpiece, activating movement of the tip

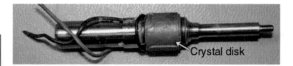

Figure 3.9 Photo of a quartz disk contained within a piezoelectric dental handpiece (Image courtesy of Dentsply Professional)

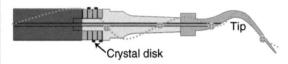

Figure 3.10 Diagram of a piezoelectric ultrasonic handpiece. Application of an alternating electrical current to the crystalline disk causes it to expand then contract, producing longitudinal vibrations that travel to the attached tip. Crosshairs denote nodal points (antinodes), or points of no movement or vibration

when subjected to an electrical field are said to be *piezoelectric* (Laird and Walmsley, 1991).

In ultrasonic dental devices with a piezoelectric transducer, an alternating electrical current is applied across a ceramic or quartz disk (Figure 3.9). In response to the alternating application of current, the crystalline structure alternatingly expands then contracts, producing vibrations that result in high-frequency oscillation of the tip (Laird and Walmsley, 1991) (Figure 3.10).

The components characteristic of a piezoelectric scaling unit are listed in Table 3.2 and illustrated by Figures 3.11–3.15.

Oscillation of tip: Stroke pattern

The direction of movement (pattern of oscillation) produced by the tip of an ultrasonic scaling instrument influences instrumentation technique, specifically how the tip of the ultrasonic instrument is adapted to the tooth.

At the time of this writing, it is generally accepted that the pattern of oscillation, commonly referred to as the *stroke pattern*, is

determined by the type of transducer, with piezoelectric scaling units producing a linear stroke pattern and magnetostrictive scaling units producing an elliptical stroke pattern.

A *linear stroke pattern* is one in which the tip of the instrument moves longitudinally forward and backward in one plane. With this linear pattern, the *kinetic energy* produced by the movement is distributed between only two surfaces of the tip – the back and the face (Figure 3.16b).

Therefore, adapting either the back or face of the tip against the tooth inherently delivers a high and potentially damaging degree of force perpendicular to the tooth surface. To avoid such undue force, it has been recommended that the lateral surfaces of a linear-movement tip be adapted to stroke parallel to the tooth surface in a sweeping-like motion.

An *elliptical stroke pattern* involves movement in multiple planes as the tip of the instrument moves longitudinally and transversely (laterally) in the shape of an oval or "ellipse" (Figure 3.16a). With this elliptical pattern, the kinetic energy produced by the movement is distributed among all surfaces – the back, face, and two lateral surfaces – of the tip.

This wide (among all surfaces) distribution of energy lessens the amount of energy directed to any one surface; therefore, any surface of an elliptical-movement tip can be adapted to the tooth without inherently exerting an overt amount of force to the tooth surface. The capacity to utilize any surface of the tip is advantageous to efficient debridement and will be addressed in greater detail in Chapter 6, Ultrasonic Instrumentation Technique.

The belief that piezoelectric scaling units produce linear stroke patterns and magnetostrictive scaling units produce elliptical stroke patterns resulted from the findings of several studies (Walmsley et al., 1986; Gankerseer and Walmsley, 1987), which utilized light microscopy (measurement of reflected light) to demonstrate the pattern of tip oscillation (Lea et al., 2002, 2009a). Since the time when these studies were conducted, newer technology has become

Table 3.2 Components of piezoelectric ultrasonic units

Component	Description
Tip	

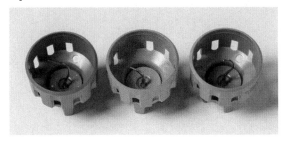

Screws onto handpiece by a torque-controlled wrench

Figure 3.11 Piezoelectric tips and tip wrenches/carriers

Handpiece

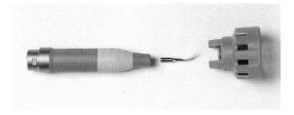

Embeds ceramic or crystal disks which encircle a metal bar. The terminal end of the bar is screw threaded to allow attachment of the tip

Figure 3.12 Handpiece of a piezoelectric unit to which the tip is attached using the torque wrench

Base unit

Houses controls which regulate power level and water flow; provides connection between foot switch and handpiece

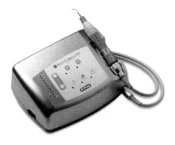

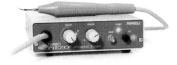

Figure 3.14 TurboPIEZO™ piezoelectric scaler (Image courtesy of Parkell, Inc.)

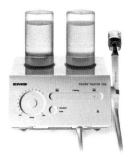

Figure 3.13 Symmetry IQ® piezoelectric scaler (Image courtesy of Hu-Friedy Mfg Co., LLC, Chicago IL, USA)

Figure 3.15 Piezon® Master 700 piezoelectric scaler (Image courtesy of Electro Medical Systems Corporation, Dallas, TX)

Foot switch — When engaged, sends electrical current through base unit to the handpiece, activating movement of the tip

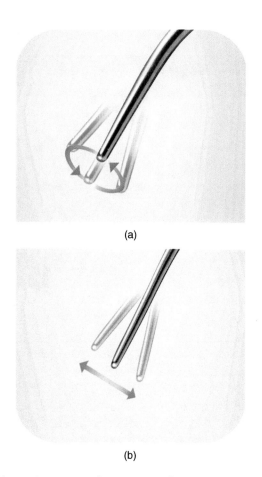

(a)

(b)

Figure 3.16 Tip oscillation in (a) an elliptical stroke pattern compared to (b) a linear stroke pattern

available which utilizes scanning laser vibrometry to measure the oscillations of ultrasonic scaler tips three-dimensionally.

Using 3D laser vibrometry, Lea et al. (2009a) evaluated the oscillation patterns of piezoelectric and magnetostrictive ultrasonic instruments in loaded (adapted to a tooth) and unloaded (oscillating freely in air) conditions at low- and high-power settings. In contrast to the findings of the light microscopy studies, this study demonstrated that both piezoelectric and magnetostrictive scaling instruments oscillate in an elliptical pattern, with the magnitude of the lateral movement varying according to tip shape and power setting. These findings were further substantiated

in a root surface defect study conducted by Lea et al. (2009b).

> ### Box 3.1: Key point
>
> Both piezoelectric and magnetostrictive tips oscillate in an elliptical pattern, with the broadness of the elliptical movement varying with power setting and tip shape.

In other words, the type of transducer, piezoelectric or magnetostrictive, does not determine the stroke pattern produced by the tip, as previously believed; both produce elliptical stroke patterns. The elliptical pattern will vary transversely from near-linear to broad depending on the power setting and tip shape. Slimmer tip shapes are more likely to produce broad elliptical movement, especially at higher power settings; low power and wider tip shapes are more likely to produce narrow (near-linear) elliptical movement (Lea et al., 2009a, 2009b). See Figures 3.17a,b and 3.18.

As stated at the beginning of this discussion on oscillation, the stroke pattern of the tip influences instrumentation technique, specifically adaptation of the ultrasonic instrument. Based on this most recent evidence (Lea et al., 2009a, b), this textbook approaches ultrasonic instrumentation technique and tip selection from the perspective that both piezoelectric and magnetostrictive instruments produce an elliptical stroke pattern.

ULTRASONIC INSTRUMENTATION MECHANISMS OF ACTION

The high-frequency vibrations induced by both magnetostrictive and piezoelectric transducers are ultimately directed to the tip of the ultrasonic instrument. High-frequency oscillation of the tip produces mechanical and biophysical forces that disrupt and remove deposits on the surface of the tooth (Walmsley et al., 2008). These forces are

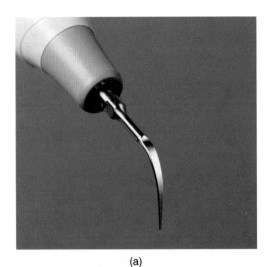

(a)

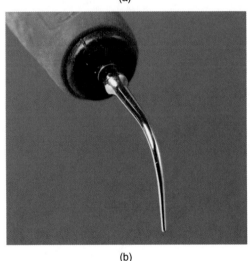

(b)

Figure 3.17 Tips designs evaluated by Lea et al., 2009a. (a) piezoelectric tip design; (b) magnetostrictive tip design. Note the broader/flatter design of the piezoelectric tip compared to the slimmer/cylindrical design of the magnetostrictive tip

considered the *mechanisms of action* by which ultrasonic instruments achieve debridement and are summarized in Table 3.3.

Mechanical

The primary mechanism of ultrasonic debridement is mechanical (Walmsley et al., 1984, 1988;

Lea et al., 2009b). The vibratory action of the oscillating metal tip against the deposit mechanically fractures or breaks the deposit from the tooth surface. Calculus removal with ultrasonic instruments generally occurs by ablation (or attrition) of the calcified deposit from the outer surface of the deposit down to the tooth surface (Figure 3.19a), but may also occur by breaking the calculus from the tooth at the tooth–deposit interface.

In contrast, manual scaling instruments and manual scaling technique are designed to break the bond between the tooth and deposit at the tooth–deposit interface (Figure 3.19b), although ablation of the deposit can also occur depending on a number of working parameters, including sharpness of the cutting edge and lateral force (Lea and Walmsley, 2009). Incomplete ablation of the calculus, whether by manual or ultrasonic instrumentation, is termed *burnished calculus*.

Irrigation

A flow of irrigant (typically water) cools the tip and creates a continuous *lavage* during instrumentation, which assists flushing of the debris from the treatment site and improving operator visibility. As the lavage extends to the full extent of the tip's penetration into the periodontal pocket (Nosal et al., 1991), the removal of loosely attached biofilm and endotoxin from the root surface by the lavage likely occurs as well. Moore et al. (1986) demonstrated that 39% of endotoxin on periodontally involved roots could be removed by a gentle, one-minute washing of the root surface, and the removal of biofilm by low-velocity fluid streams with entrapped air bubbles has been demonstrated *in vitro* (Parini et al., 2005).

Cavitation and acoustic microstreaming

As the cooling water flows over the oscillating tip, ultrasonic energy is imparted into the water,

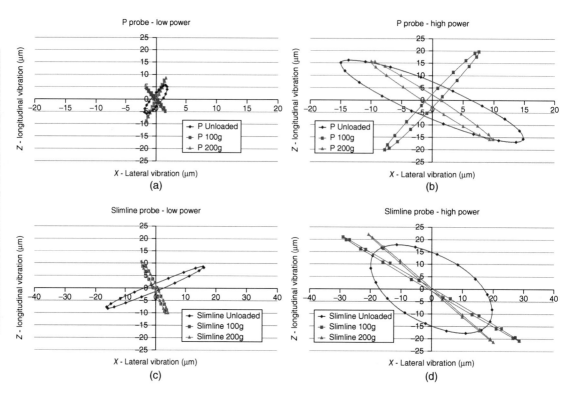

Figure 3.18 Oscillation patterns of loaded and unloaded P (broad/flat) and Slimline (slim/cylindrical) tips at high- and low-generator powers. Both tip designs demonstrate elliptical motion under load. Plots show P tip at (a) low power and (b) high power, and Slimline tip at (c) low power and (d) high power. Axes show probe displacement amplitudes measured in micrometer (*Source:* Lea et al., 2009a. Reproduced with permission of John Wiley & Sons, Inc.)

Table 3.3 Ultrasonic debridement mechanisms of action

Mechanical	Vibratory action of the oscillating metal tip against the deposit ablates/breaks the deposit from the tooth surface
Irrigation	Lavage action of water flowing over tip flushes biofilm from the tooth surface and debris from the treatment site
Cavitation	Removal/disruption of biofilm by shock waves resulting from the implosion of bubbles
Acoustic microstreaming	Removal/disruption of biofilm by turbulent currents of water surrounding the tip

generating two biophysical forces which likely contribute to the removal of biofilm – cavitation and acoustic microstreaming (Walmsley et al., 1992).

Cavitation is a hydrodynamic occurrence that can be defined as the formation and subsequent implosion of pulsating cavities, or "bubbles" in a flowing liquid that is the consequence of forces acting on the liquid (Laird and Walmsley, 1991). The bubbles are filled with water vapor/gas, so the implosion of the bubbles radiates shock waves or high-velocity liquid jets that have the ability to remove strongly bound particulate matter from solid surfaces (Walmsley et al., 1984, 1985; Laird and Walmsley, 1991). Figure 3.20 illustrates the occurrence of cavitation.

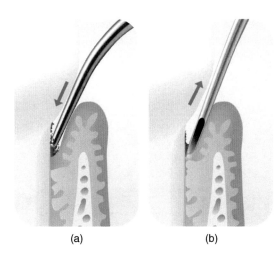

(a)   (b)

Figure 3.19 Calculus removal by (a) ablation or attrition of the calcified deposit from the outer surface of the calculus down to the tooth surface versus (b) breaking of the calculus from the tooth at the tooth–deposit interface

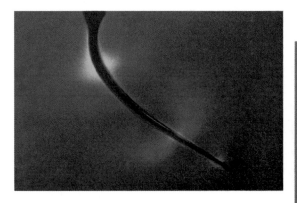

Figure 3.21 Luminol photography of an ultrasonic scaling tip at power 10/10. Light regions indicate areas of high-cavitation activity, with dark regions indicating little or no activity (*Source*: Felver et al., 2009. Reproduced with permission from Elsevier)

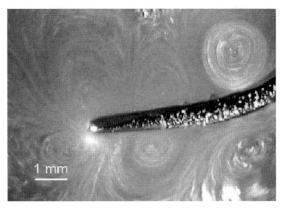

Figure 3.22 Video captured digitized image of a magnetostrictive insert (P-12) showing acoustic microstreaming as demonstrated by the movement of zinc stearate particles floating on the water surface into which the scaler tip is oscillating at 10.5 μm displacement amplitude (*Source*: Khambay and Walmsley, 1999. Reproduced with permission of American Academy of Periodontology)

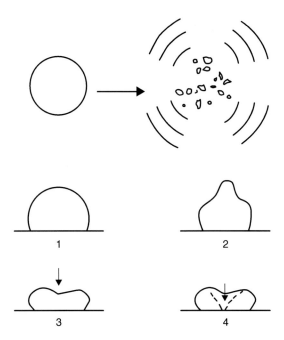

1   2

3   4

Figure 3.20 Diagrammatic representation of a free bubble collapsing to smaller fragments and radiating shock waves. (1) bubble on solid surface; (2) undergoing deformation; (3) producing a high- velocity liquid jet; (4) jet pierces bubble and damages solid surface (*Source*: Laird et al., 1991. Reproduced with permission of Elsevier)

Cavitation does occur within the cooling water surrounding the oscillating ultrasonic scaler tip (Walmsley et al., 1984, 1986; Lea et al., 2005; Felver et al., 2009), as illustrated in Figure 3.21.

Acoustic microstreaming is a phenomenon characterized by small-scale ("micro") vigorous circulatory motion of fluid. Microstreaming occurs near any object in oscillatory motion, including sonic or ultrasonic scaler tips (Figure 3.22) and pulsating cavitation bubbles (Nyborg, 1977; Khambay and Walmsley, 1999).

WHAT IS ULTRASONIC INSTRUMENTATION?

This vigorous, yet low-velocity, current of fluid produces hydrodynamic shearing forces in close proximity to the oscillating scaler tip or gas bubble (Nyborg, 1977; Khambay and Walmsley, 1999). These shear forces are strong enough to disrupt or damage biological cells (Nyborg, 1977) and have demonstrated efficacy in removing a dental plaque substitute from a glass slide (Khambay and Walmsley, 1999), indicating that acoustic microstreaming may likely play a role in the disruption and removal of biofilm and loosely attached deposits from tooth surfaces.

Cavitation and acoustic microstreaming are related and synergistic in their mechanisms of action (Khambay and Walmsley, 1999). The combined effect of the cavitational and microstreaming forces extends biofilm removal up to 0.5 mm distant from the area of tooth contacted by the oscillating tip, following the path of the cooling water as it flows over and away from the tip (Figure 3.23) (Walmsley et al., 1988).

These findings are evidence that the efficacy of ultrasonic instrumentation in the disruption and removal of biofilm is not only a result of the mechanical action of the oscillating tip, but is also enhanced by the biophysical forces generated within the cooling water surrounding the tip (Walmsley et al., 1988).

ULTRASONIC SCALER OPERATIONAL VARIABLES

Operational variables common to all oscillating scaling technologies – sonic and ultrasonic magnetostrictive and piezoelectric – include operating frequency, power setting, and water flow rate (Table 3.4).

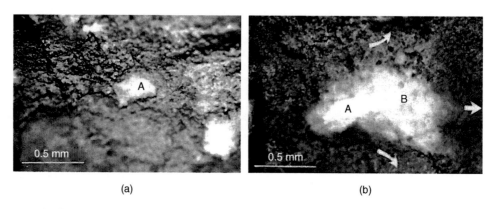

(a)   (b)

Figure 3.23 The dark area on the photomicrograph is the stained dental plaque. Plaque removal by the (a) nonwater and (b) water cooled sickle scaling tip oscillating at 31 μm. In both images, plaque is removed by the vibratory action of the tip (area A). Additional removal (area B) resulting from cavitational activity is seen in image (b). The direction of water flow is indicated by arrows (*Source*: Walmsley et al., 1988. Reproduced with permission of John Wiley & Sons, Inc.)

Table 3.4 Ultrasonic scaler operational variables

Frequency	The number of back and forth strokes the tip oscillates per second, measured in kilohertz (kHz). Typically fixed at resonate frequency of 30 or 25 kHz.
Power input (setting)	Adjusts the length of the strokes (displacement amplitude) of the oscillating tip, thereby influencing the amount of force and cavitation generated by the tip.
Water flow rate	Adjusts the amount of water (or other irrigant) flowing through the handpiece and over the oscillating tip.

Operating frequency

Frequency is defined as the rate at which something occurs or is repeated within a specific period of time. For an oscillating object then, frequency is the number of complete back and forth cycles per second. Specific to ultrasonic scaling equipment, the *operating frequency* of the unit is the number of strokes the oscillating tip completes per second.

The standard unit of measurement of frequency is hertz, abbreviated Hz. If an object oscillates 1 cycle per second, then the frequency is 1 Hz; 100 cycles per second equals 100 Hz. A larger unit of frequency is the kilohertz (kHz), which represents thousands of cycles per second.

Typical operating frequencies of contemporary ultrasonic scaling units are 30 kHz (magnetostrictive and piezoelectric) or 25 kHz (magnetostrictive). Therefore, tips operating at 30 kHz are completing 30,000 elliptical strokes per second.

A *resonant frequency* is a natural frequency of vibration determined by the physical parameters of the vibrating object. For example, each string on a guitar, when plucked, will vibrate at its resonate frequency as determined by the length, mass, and tension of the string, that is, its physical parameters. This resonate frequency consistently produces the pitch unique to that string.

Similarly, ultrasonic scaling units are manufactured to oscillate at a resonate frequency, enabling optimal tip vibration with minimal power requirements (Lea and Walmsley, 2009). The unit is locked into the resonate frequency of the transducer and adjustment of the frequency by the clinician is not possible. The term *auto-tuned* is sometimes used in reference to scaling units operating at a locked resonate frequency.

There are a minority of clinicians advocating the use of *manual-tuned* ultrasonic scaling units, which allow adjustment of the operating frequency in an attempt to improve patient comfort or improve operator visibility during endoscopic periodontal debridement (Kwan, 2005). Changing the operating frequency of a scaling unit from the resonate frequency – which ensures optimal performance – reduces the efficiency of deposit removal, thereby increasing the working time required to complete thorough instrumentation.

Power input

While the number of oscillating strokes produced per second by an ultrasonic scaling unit is typically fixed, the length of the oscillating strokes produced is variable.

The range of movement, or the stroke length, of the oscillating tip is measured as the *displacement amplitude*, that is, how far the tip is displaced from a position of zero movement. The displacement amplitude of ultrasonic scaling tips is measured in microns (µm), 1 µm being equivalent to 0.001 mm, and represents half the peak to peak displacement of the tip (Walmsley et al., 1986). Figure 3.24 illustrates the displacement amplitude.

The maximum displacement amplitude occurs at the free, unconstrained end of the oscillating tip and is influenced by both the amount of power supplied to the transducer and the design of the scaling tip (Walmsley et al., 1986; Lea et al., 2003a, 2009a, 2009b; Felver et al., 2009; Walmsley et al., 2013).

Influence of power input on displacement amplitude

The *power setting* of the unit can be adjusted to vary the amount of electrical power input to the transducer. Increasing the electrical power input to the transducer increases the displacement amplitude of the tip, lengthening the stroke; decreasing the power input to the transducer decreases the displacement amplitude of the tip, shortening the stroke (Walmsley et al., 1986; Chapple et al., 1995). (Figure 3.25)

Because of this positive, but not necessarily linear, correlation between power input and displacement amplitude, the power level can function as an estimate of the stroke length produced (Lea et al., 2003a). Contemporary ultrasonic scaling devices are designed to arbitrarily estimate the power level using a linear scale ranging from low to high power (Figure 3.26), as opposed to accurately measuring the displacement amplitude of the oscillating tip in microns.

Influence of tip design on displacement amplitude

However, the extent to which the power input increases or decreases the displacement amplitude is variable and dependent on the design of the scaling tip. At the same power setting, different tip designs, as well as different tips of the same design, will oscillate with different displacement amplitudes (Walmsley et al., 1986; Gankerseer and Walmsley, 1987; Trenter et al., 2003; Lea et al., 2002, 2003a, 2003b, 2006, 2009a, 2009b).

The clinical significance of this variability is that, in order to achieve the same level of performance, different power settings are required for different tips (Lea et al., 2003a); therefore, clinicians should expect to make adjustments to the power setting for each tip utilized in practice.

It is also important to understand that standardization of power input settings does not exist between types of generators (piezoelectric or magnetostrictive) or between manufacturers of the same type of generators. Studies have demonstrated greater displacement amplitudes (Lea et al., 2003a), and thereby greater root surface damage (Busslinger et al., 2001), from piezoelectric devices compared to magnetostrictive devices operating at the same power settings with tips of similar design. This inherent variability in power settings requires adjustments to the power input as appropriate in consideration of the type of generator, as well as tip design and type of deposit.

Water flow rate

Contact between the high-frequency oscillating tip and the tooth surface can generate an increase in temperature referred to as *frictional heating* (Walmsley and Williams, 1986; Lea et al., 2004). This heat can be absorbed by the dental tissues and results in an elevated tooth temperature (Walmsley and Williams, 1986).

To minimize the production of frictional heat, all ultrasonic instruments are operated with a continuous supply of water flowing over the oscillating tip to act as a coolant. As the water flows over the tip–tooth interface, the heat generated is conducted into the water and carried

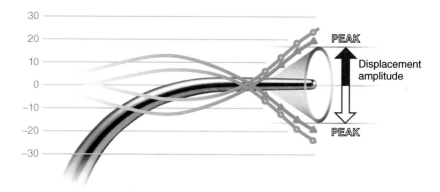

Figure 3.24 Plotting the maximum vibration along the length of the scaler tip (values shown are the mean of 10 readings ± 1 standard deviation) demonstrates how far the tip is displaced from a position of zero movement. Displacement amplitude is measured as half the peak to peak displacement of the tip and is greatest at the free, unconstrained end of the oscillating tip (*Source*: Lea et al., 2009b. Modified with permission of Sage Publications)

WHAT IS ULTRASONIC INSTRUMENTATION?

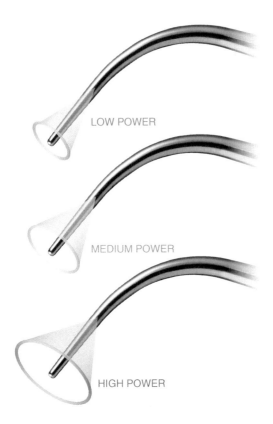

Figure 3.25 Effect of power setting on displacement amplitude (stroke length) of tip

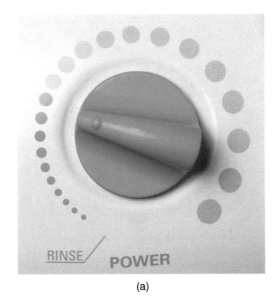

(a)

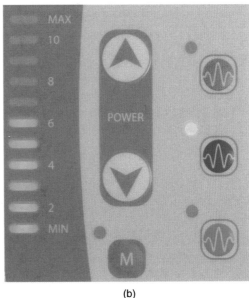

(b)

Figure 3.26 Arbitrary power input control dials of contemporary (a) magnetostrictive and (b) piezoelectric scaling units

away by the bulk fluid movement (Walmsley and Williams, 1986; Lea et al., 2004). In magnetostrictive units, the water also flows over and cools the stack of nickel strips.

During operation, frictional heat will be produced if the amount of water flowing over the tip is insufficient, whether due to an inadequate flow rate or aerosolization of the water. *Aerosolization* results from high power settings, which cause the water to be thrown off the tip as a fine mist before it reaches the working end of the tip (Figure 3.27), thereby providing no heat regulation (Lea et al., 2002).

An adequate supply of water to the tip is also essential for the generation of a lavage and the biophysical forces of cavitation and acoustic microstreaming. Under normal operating conditions, a flow rate of 20–30 ml/min provides a sufficient amount of water for cooling (Walmsley and Williams, 1986; Kocher and Plagmann, 1996; Nicoll and Peters, 1998; Trenter and Walmsley, 2003) and the occurrence of cavitation and microstreaming (Walmsley et al., 1984, 1986, 1988, 1990; Walmsley and Williams, 1986).

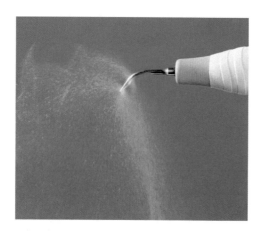

Figure 3.27 Aerosolization of the cooling water resulting from a high power setting

As with displacement amplitude, tip design and power input also influence the amount of water produced by the oscillating tip. The amount of water emitted varies among tips of different designs as well as among tips of the same design (Lea et al., 2002; Koster et al., 2009). Higher power settings atomize the water creating an aerosol, whereas lower power settings typically result in a steady stream of water that flows over the length of the tip (Lea et al., 2002). Because

of this variability in water flow rate, the clinician should expect to make adjustments to the water flow rate for each tip utilized in practice.

Currently, the water flow rate control on ultrasonic scaling units does not specify an exact measurement (ml/min) of the flow produced; rather, it provides an arbitrary estimate of the flow rate ranging from low to high (Koster et al., 2009) (Figure 3.28).

Typically, a flow rate that effectively cools and maximizes cavitation and microstreaming activity is one that produces intermittent droplets at the activated tip (Figure 3.29). To generate this effective flow rate, a medium power level should be selected and the water flow control adjusted until droplets are intermittently released from the tip.

This recommendation to produce droplets at the tip is evidence-based and in contrast to instrumentation guidelines suggesting the production of a fine mist or halo at the tip (Nield-Gehrig, 2008). As just discussed, a fine mist is insufficient to regulate the generation of frictional heat (Lea et al., 2002). Additionally, such an inadequate supply of water to the oscillating tip consequently reduces the occurrence of

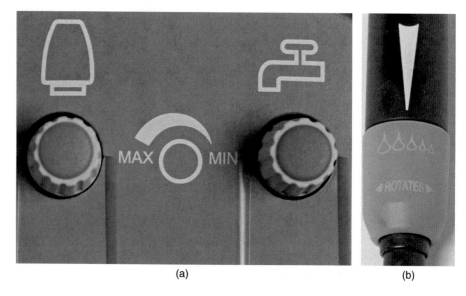

(a)   (b)

Figure 3.28 Arbitrary water flow rate control dials of contemporary (a) piezoelectric and (b) magnetostrictive scaling units

cavitation and microstreaming and the surface area debrided (Walmsley et al., 1988).

ACOUSTIC POWER OF THE ULTRASONIC SCALER

It is the combined actions of these operational variables – frequency, displacement amplitude, and water flow rate – which synergistically determine the overall *acoustic power* produced by the ultrasonic scaler.

The acoustic power emitted by the ultrasonic scaler is a product of (a) the efficiency of the mechanical mechanism of action and (b) the amount of cavitational and microstreaming activity, both of which can be accurately measured by the displacement amplitude (Walmsley et al., 1986).

Efficiency of mechanical mechanism of action

The efficiency of the vibrating tip in fracturing calculus deposits from the tooth surface correlates to the amount of force exerted by the tip. The more force exerted by the tip, the more efficiently the calculus will fracture.

Per Newton's Second Law of Motion, a degree of force results when an object, such as the ultrasonic scaling tip, is accelerated or decelerated in a certain direction. The net *force* (F) of the object is a product of the object's mass (m) multiplied by its acceleration (a) (Hewitt, 1997). See Figure 3.30.

Acceleration of a moving object (i.e., the oscillating ultrasonic tip) is influenced by distance and calculated by dividing the distance by the square of time (Hewitt, 1997). The distance in this calculation is the displacement amplitude of the oscillating tip.

Therefore, when the mass of the object remains constant, an increase in distance will increase the acceleration of the object, resulting in an increase in the net force exerted by the object. In other

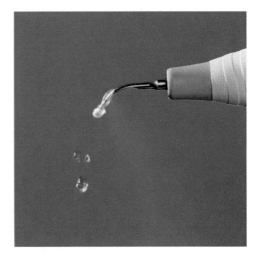

Figure 3.29 An effective flow rate demonstrated by the production of intermittent droplets at the activated tip at a medium power setting

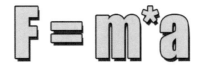

Figure 3.30 Newton's Second Law of Motion. Net force equals mass multiplied by acceleration

words, the greater the displacement amplitude, the greater the force exerted by the oscillating tip (Figure 3.31).

The influence of an object's mass on the magnitude of force exerted is addressed in Chapter 4; Insert/Tip Design and Criteria for Selection.

Given the influence of displacement amplitude on force, the displacement amplitude of the oscillating tip can affect scaling efficiency, as just described, as well as the degree of root surface damage. Increasing levels of power (i.e., increasing displacement amplitudes) result in an increase in loss of root substance or root roughness (Lie and Leknes, 1985; Flemmig et al., 1998a, 1998b; Folwaczny et al., 2004; Lea et al., 2009b).

Flemmig et al. assessed the effect of various working parameters – including low, medium and high power settings – on the depth and

Table 3.5 Influence of power setting on root surface defect depth and volume

	Magnetostrictive[1]	**Piezoelectric[2]**
Defect depth (μm)		
Low power	63.4 ± 5.2	47.9 ± 4.0
Medium power	82.5 ± 7.2	66.8 ± 5.7
High power	99.6 ± 9.1	84.5 ± 7.9
Defect volume (mm³)		
Low power	0.19 ± 0.02	0.12 ± 0.015
Medium power	0.29 ± 0.03	0.21 ± 0.028
High power	0.33 ± 0.03	0.291 ± 0.036

[1] Data obtained from Flemmig et al. (1998b)
[2] Data obtained from Flemmig et al. (1998a)

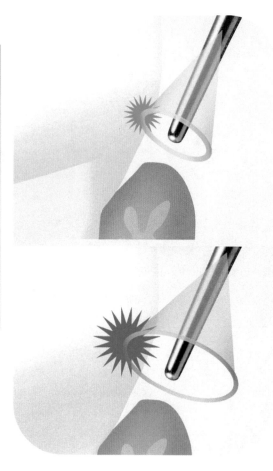

Figure 3.31 An increase in displacement amplitude results in an increase in the net force exerted by the tip

Amount of cavitational and microstreaming activity

The amount of cavitation and microstreaming activity that occurs in the cooling water surrounding the oscillating tip is relative to the overall acoustic power, as it influences both the efficiency and efficacy of biofilm debridement.

As tip displacement increases, there is a correlated increase in both cavitation (Lea et al., 2005; Felver et al., 2009; Walmsley et al., 2013) and microstreaming (Khambay and Walmsley, 1999) activity. However, the extent to which the displacement amplitude increases or decreases the amount of cavitation and microstreaming generated is influenced by the design of the scaling tip, with wider diameter/rectangular cross section tips typically producing greater cavitational and streaming forces than slim diameter/cylindrical cross section tips (Walmsley et al., 1988; Khambay and Walmsley, 1999; Lea et al., 2005; Felver et al., 2009).

Tips oscillate in a sequence of nodes and antinodes, with the maximum displacement amplitude occurring at the free, unconstrained end of the oscillating tip. Accordingly, the greatest shear microstreaming forces are in the immediate vicinity of the tip (Khambay and Walmsley, 1999). However, maximum cavitation occurs further up

volume of root surface defects following instrumentation by magnetostrictive (1998b) and piezoelectric (1998a) ultrasonic scalers. Table 3.5 summarizes the data from these studies, which shows that as power level increased, so, too, did the amount of root surface that was removed, whether measured by defect depth or volume.

Lea et al. (2009b) conducted a similar assessment of working parameters on the shape, depth, and volume of root surface defects produced by slim-diameter magnetostrictive and piezoelectric tips. In alignment with the findings of Flemmig et al. an increase in power resulted in increased displacement amplitudes as well as an increase in the depth and volume of root surface defects for both types of slim diameter tips.

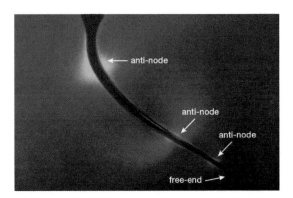

Figure 3.32 Luminol photography of an unloaded ultrasonic scaling tip at power 10/10. Light regions indicate areas of high-cavitation activity, with dark regions indicating little or no activity. Note that in unloaded conditions, the areas of high-cavitation activity occur at the vibration anti-node as opposed to the free end of the tip (*Source*: Felver et al., 2009. Reproduced with permission from Elsevier)

the unloaded oscillating tip at a vibration antinode (Felver et al., 2009; Walmsley et al., 2013) (Figure 3.32).

In order to be clinically beneficial in the debridement of biofilm from root surfaces, cavitation needs to occur at lower power settings and maximize at the free end of the tip. Walmsley et al. (2012) have demonstrated that the lateral pressure applied to maintain contact of the tip to the tooth influences cavitational activity. At lower power settings, the amount of cavitation generated increases with loads up to 2.0 N. Load also changes the distribution of the cavitational activity, from primarily at the antinode, to more occurring at the clinically useful active area of the tip, and more so with slim diameter than wide diameter tips (Walmsley et al., 2013). See Figure 3.33.

As cavitational and streaming forces increase, an increase in the surface area debrided by these forces results, with the extent of biofilm removed differing according to the orientation of the tip to the tooth (Walmsley et al., 1988; Khambay and Walmsley, 1999). Vertical adaptation of the tip to the tooth surface (adapted like a periodontal probe) resulted in an eightfold increase in biofilm removal, compared to a sixfold increase when

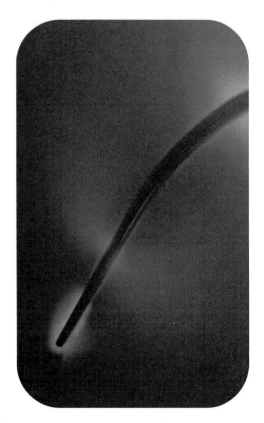

Figure 3.33 Simulation of the effect of loading on an ultrasonic scaling tip at power 10/10. Application of load shifts the distribution of cavitation, resulting in increased cavitational activity at the active area of the tip (*Source*: Felver et al., 2009. Modified with permission from Elsevier)

the tip was oriented oblique to the tooth surface (adapted like a sickle scaler) (Walmsley et al., 1988). See Figure 3.34a,b.

A synopsis of the correlational relationship between key operating variables and mechanisms of acoustic power is presented in Table 3.6.

CONCEPT OF MINIMUM EFFECTIVE POWER

While a greater displacement amplitude (higher power setting) is desirable for efficient removal of deposits (increased force for efficient calculus removal and increased cavitation for efficient

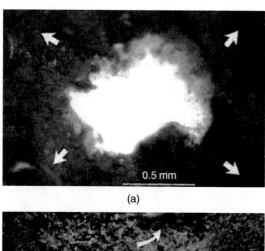

(a)

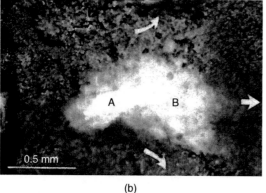

(b)

Figure 3.34 Plaque removal by tip and cavitational activity resulting from (a) vertical adaptation of the tip and (b) oblique adaptation of the tip. The direction of water flow is indicated by arrows (*Source*: Walmsley et al., 1988. Reproduced with permission of John Wiley & Sons, Inc.)

biofilm removal), a lesser displacement amplitude (lower power setting) is imperative to avoid over-instrumentation and minimize root surface damage. To meet this objective, it is then essential for the clinician to operate the ultrasonic scaling device at the *minimum effective power for the task at hand* – high enough to efficiently disrupt the deposits, but low enough to prevent or minimize damage to the root surface.

The minimum effective power required will vary according to the type of deposit to be removed (*task at hand*) and the type of generator and design of tip utilized. In general, higher power levels are needed for efficient scaling of firmly attached calculus deposits, whereas lower power levels suffice for the debridement of biofilm and light calculus. Remarkably, the threshold power level for root surface debridement, that is, the stroke length at which the greatest amount of cavitation is produced without inherently over-instrumenting the root surface, appears to be in the range of a medium power setting (Lie and Leknes, 1985; Baehni et al., 1987; Walmsley et al., 1988; Jacobson et al., 1994; Flemmig et al., 1998a, 1998b; Lea et al., 2005; Felver et al., 2009; Walmsley et al., 2013), rather than perhaps a more presumable low power setting.

Utilization of a minimum effective power approach to ultrasonic instrumentation achieves

Table 3.6 Relationship of ultrasonic operating variables and mechanisms of acoustic power

Variable	Displacement amplitude (DA)	Cavitation (CA) and microstreaming (AMS)	Force (F)
Power input	+ correlation ↑ electrical input = ↑DA	+ correlation ↑ electrical input = ↑ DA = ↑ CA/AMS	+ correlation ↑ electrical input = ↑DA = ↑F
Tip diameter	Variable	+ correlation ↑ tip diameter = ↑ CA/AMS	+ correlation ↑ tip diameter = ↑F
Water flow at tip	– correlation High DA = fine mist	+ correlation ↑ water at tip = ↑CA/AMS	

periodontal healing while minimizing root surface damage. The use of a medium power setting has been demonstrated to be as effective as a high power setting in achieving periodontal healing, as measured by standard clinical indices (Chapple et al., 1995). Therefore, operating the ultrasonic scaler consistently at a higher power setting under the assumption of improved scaling and debridement efficiency or efficacy cannot be justified (Box 3.2).

Box 3.2: Key point

Although ultrasonic scaling units allow for a wide range of power input (low to high), evidence suggests that a more limited range of power, medium to medium–high, may be all that is necessary to achieve effective periodontal debridement.

Guidelines for the selection of appropriate power setting and other working parameters are provided Chapter 6, Stages of Ultrasonic Instrumentation.

SONIC SCALING TECHNOLOGY

Sonic, or air turbine, scaling devices operate at a lower frequency of vibration than ultrasonic scaling devices, typically in the sonic range of 16–18 kHz (Gankerseer and Walmsley, 1987) (Figure 3.1). The *sonic scaler* is attached directly to an air handpiece coupler on the dental unit (Figure 3.35). Oscillation of the tip results from the passage of air over a metal rod contained within the handpiece of the instrument

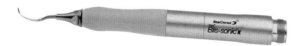

Figure 3.35 Titan® Blis-sonic™ sonic scaler (Image courtesy of DentalEZ Group)

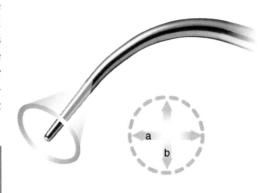

Figure 3.36 Elliptical oscillation of the sonic scaler, with (a) transverse movement being ≥ (b) longitudinal movement

(Gankerseer and Walmsley, 1987). As with ultrasonic scaling devices, cooling water runs through the handpiece to the oscillating tip to reduce the occurrence of frictional heat.

The pattern of tip oscillation for the sonic scaler is elliptical (Figure 3.36), with the transverse movement being at least as large as the longitudinal movement (Gankerseer and Walmsley, 1987; Jacobsen et al., 1994).

Displacement amplitude

The displacement amplitude of the oscillating sonic tip is influenced by air pressure input, tip design, and load. As with ultrasonic scalers, displacement amplitude varies with tip design, but is more easily dampened by higher load compared to ultrasonic scalers, which may interfere with tip oscillation (Gankerseer and Walmsley, 1987; Ritz et al., 1991).

A significant limitation of the sonic scaling device is that displacement amplitude of the tip cannot be adjusted by the clinician; instead it is determined by the air pressure input into the handpiece, an operational variable not easily manipulated in the clinical environment. Gankerseer and Walmsley (1987) demonstrated that increasing air pressure input increased the displacement amplitude, with the greatest increase in amplitude occurring in the transverse direction. Clinically, the inability of the clinician to decrease the displacement amplitude is more of a concern than the inability to increase it, as the sonic scaler inherently oscillates at large amplitude, which is destructive to the root surface. Because of the significant increase in root surface loss resulting from sonic scalers compared to ultrasonic scalers (Chapter 2), the use of the sonic scaler is contraindicated for root surface debridement and limited to coronal scaling. To take full advantage of the mechanisms of sonic scaling, the clinician should utilize the sonic instrument following the principles of technique outlined in Chapter 6.

RECENT DEVELOPMENTS IN ULTRASONIC TECHNOLOGY

The desire to further reduce root surface alteration during ultrasonic instrumentation has led to the development of a novel ultrasonic device which oscillates linearly, but in a vertical (up and down) direction, as opposed to the longitudinal (forward and backward) linear stroke pattern defined earlier in this chapter. This vertical stroke pattern allows the tip to oscillate parallel to the tooth surface, eliminating any transverse (elliptical) vibrations against the tooth, resulting in significantly less removal of root substance than a conventional ultrasonic system (Rupf et al., 2005; Kawashima et al., 2007).

The ultrasonic vibrations are generated by a piezoelectric transducer, but are transmitted via a flexible ring to a working tip that is positioned 90° to the instrument handpiece (Figure 3.37) to facilitate the vertical motion (Guentsch and Preshaw, 2008; Lea and Walmsley, 2009).

Because the vertical stroke pattern diminishes the mechanical (vibratory) mechanism of deposit

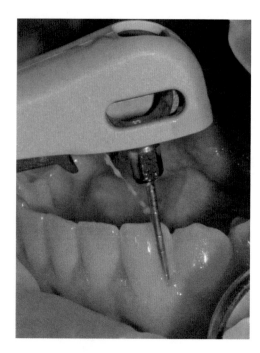

Figure 3.37 The Vector™ system (Image courtesy of Dr. Arndt Güentsch, University of Jena, Germany)

removal, using the device in conjunction with abrasive and polishing fluids is necessary to accomplish effective scaling and debridement (Braun et al., 2006). The occurrence of cavitation around this type of device has not been evaluated to date (Lea and Walmsley, 2009).

Several papers reviewing the efficacy of this novel approach to ultrasonic debridement have determined that, while use of the device results in clinical outcomes comparable to those achieved by traditional ultrasonic instruments (Guentsch and Preshaw, 2008; Walmsley et al., 2008), treatment is more time consuming than conventional debridement (Braun et al., 2006) and is not effective in removing heavy calculus deposits (Guentsch and Preshaw, 2008). As the vertical oscillations are less damaging than the elliptical oscillations of conventional ultrasonic instruments, use of this device may be advantageous for periodontal maintenance and implant maintenance procedures (Guentsch and Preshaw, 2008).

REFERENCES

Braun A, Krause F, Hartschen V, Falk W, Jepsen S. Efficiency of the Vector™- system compared with conventional subgingival debridement in vitro and in vivo. *J Clin Periodontol* 2006; 33: 568–74.

Busslinger A, Lampe K, Buechat M, Lehmann B. A comparative in vitro study of a magnetostrictive and a piezoelectric ultrasonic scaling instrument. *J Clin Periodontol* 2001; 28: 642–9.

Chapple ILC, Walmsley AD, Sasby MS, Moscrop H. Effect of instrument power setting during ultrasonic scaling upon treatment outcome. *J Periodontol* 1995; 66: 756–60.

Christgau M, Manner T, Beuer S, Hiller KA, Schmalz G. Periodontal healing after non-surgical therapy with a modified sonic scaler: a controlled clinical trial. *J Periodontol* 2006; 33: 749–58.

Felver B, King DC, Lea SC, Price GJ, Walmsley AD. Cavitation occurrence around ultrasonic dental scalers. *Ultrason Sonochem* 2009; 16: 692–7.

Flemmig TF, Petersilka GJ, Mehl A, Hickel R, Klaiber B. The effect of working parameters on root substance removal using a piezoelectric ultrasonic scaler in vitro. *J Clin Periodontol* 1998a; 25: 158–63.

Flemmig TF, Petersilka GJ, Mehl A, Hickel R, Klaiber B. Working parameters of a magnetostrictive ultrasonic scaler influencing root substance removal in vitro. *J Periodontol* 1998b; 69: 547–53.

Folwaczny M, Merkel U, Mehl A, Hickel R. Influence of parameters on root surface roughness following treatment with a magnetostrictive ultrasonic scaler: an in vitro study. *J Periodontol* 2004; 75: 1221–6.

Gankerseer EJ, Walmsley AD. Preliminary investigation into the performance of a sonic scaler. *J Periodontol* 1987; 58: 780–4.

Guentsch A, Preshaw PM. The use of a linear oscillating device in periodontal treatment: a review. *J Clin Periodontol* 2008; 35: 514–24.

Hewitt PG. *Conceptual physics.* 3rd edn. Boston: Addison-Wesley Publishing Company; 1997.

Jacobson L, Blomlof J, Lindskog S. Root surface texture after different scaling modalities. *Scan J Dent Res* 1994; 102: 156–60.

Kawashima H, Sato S, Kishida M, Ito K. A comparison of root surface instrumentation using two piezoelectric ultrasonic scalers and a hand scaler in vivo. *J Periodontal Res* 2007; 42: 90–5.

Khambay BS, Walmsley AD. Acoustic microstreaming: detection and measurement around ultrasonic scalers. *J Periodontol* 1999; 70: 626–31.

Kocher T, Plagmann HC. Heat propagation in dentin during instrumentation with different sonic scaler tips. *Quintessence Int* 1996; 27: 259–64.

Koster TJG, Timmerman MF, Feilzer AJ, Van der Velden U, Van der Weijden FA. Water coolant supply in relation to different ultrasonic scaler systems, tips and coolant settings. *J Clin Periodontol* 2009; 36: 127–31.

Kwan JY. Enhanced periodontal debridement with the use of micro ultrasonic, periodontal endoscopy. *J Calif Dent Assoc* 2005; 33: 241–8.

Laird WRE, Walmsley AD. Ultrasound in dentistry. Part 1 - biophysical interactions. *J Dent* 1991; 19: 14–7.

Laurell L, Pettersson B. Periodontal healing after treatment with either the Titan-S sonic scaler or hand instruments. *Swed Dent J* 1988; 12: 187–92.

Lea SC, Felver B, Landini G, Walmsley AD. Three-dimensional analyses of ultrasonic scaler oscillations. *J Clin Periodontol* 2009a; 36: 44–50.

Lea SC, Felver B, Landini G, Walmsley AD. Ultrasonic scaler oscillations and tooth-surface defects. *J Dent Res* 2009b; 88: 229–34.

Lea SC, Landini G, Walmsley AD. Vibration characteristics of ultrasonic scalers assessed with scanning laser vibrometry. *J Dent* 2002; 30: 147–51.

Lea SC, Landini G, Walmsley AD. Displacement amplitude of ultrasonic scaler inserts. *J Clin Periodontol* 2003a; 30: 505–10.

Lea SC, Landini G, Walmsley AD. Ultrasonic scaler tip performance under various load conditions. *J Clin Periodontol* 2003b; 30: 876–81.

Lea SC, Landini G, Walmsley AD. Thermal imaging of ultrasonic scaler tips during tooth instrumentation. *J Clin Periodontol* 2004; 31: 370–5.

Lea SC, Landini G, Walmsley AD. The effect of tip wear on ultrasonic scaler tip displacement amplitude. *J Clin Periodontol* 2006; 33: 37–41.

Lea SC, Price GJ, Walmsley AD. A study to determine whether cavitation occurs around dental ultrasonic scaling instruments. *Ultrason Sonochem* 2005; 12: 233–6.

Lea SC, Walmsley AD. Mechano-physical and biophysical properties of power-driven scalers: driving the future of powered instrument design and evaluation. *Periodontol 2000* 2009; 51: 63–78.

Lie T, Leknes KN. Evaluation of the effect on root surfaces of air turbine scalers and ultrasonic instrumentation. *J Periodontol* 1985; 56: 522–31.

Loos B, Kiger R, Egelberg J. An evaluation of basic periodontal therapy using sonic and ultrasonic scalers. *J Clin Periodontol* 1987; 14: 29–33.

Moore J, Wilson M, Kieser JB. The distribution of bacterial lipopolysaccharide (endotoxin) in relation to periodontally involved root surfaces. *J Clin Periodontol* 1986; 13: 748–51.

Nicoll BK, Peters RJ. Heat generation during ultrasonic instrumentation of dentin as affected by different irrigation methods. *J Periodontol* 1988; 69: 884–8.

Nield-Gehrig, JS. *Fundamentals of periodontal instrumentation & advanced root instrumentation*. Baltimore: Lippincott Williams & Wilkins; 2008.

Nosal G, Scheidt MJ, O'Neal R, Van Dyke TE. The penetration of lavage solution into the periodontal pocket during ultrasonic instrumentation. *J Periodontol* 1991; 62: 554–7.

Nyborg WL (1977). *Physical Mechanisms for Biological Effects of Ultrasound*. Washington, DC: HEW Publication(FDA) pp. 77–80.

Obeid PR, D'Hoore W, Bercy P. Comparative clinical responses related to the use of various periodontal instrumentation. *J Clin Periodontol* 2004; 31: 193–9.

Oda S, Nitta H, Setoguchi T, Izumi Y, Ishikawa I. Current concepts and advances in manual and power-driven instrumentation. *Periodontol 2000* 2004; 36: 45–58.

Parini MR, Eggett DL, Pitt WG. Removal of Streptococcus mutans biofilm by bubbles. *J Clin Periodontol* 2005; 32: 1151–6.

Ritz L, Hefti AF, Rateitschak KH. An in vitro investigation on the loss of root substance in scaling with various instruments. *J Clin Periodontol* 1991; 18: 643–7.

Rupf S, Brader I, Vonderlind D, Kannengiesser S, Eschrich K, Roeder I et al., In vitro, clinical, and microbiological evaluation of a linear oscillating device for scaling and root planing. *J Periodontol* 2005; 76: 1942–9.

Thilo BE, Baehni PC. Effect of ultrasonic instrumentation on dental plaque microflora in vitro. *J Periodont Res* 1987; 22: 518–21.

Trenter SC, Landini G, Walmsley AD. Effect of loading on the vibration characteristics of thin magnetostrictive ultrasonic scaler inserts. *J Periodontol* 2003; 74: 1308–15.

Trenter SC, Walmsley AD. Ultrasonic dental scaler: associated hazards. *J Clin Periodontol* 2003; 30: 95–101.

Walmsley AD. Ultrasonic and sonic scalers. *Br Dent Surg Assist* 1989; 48: 26–8.

Walmsley AD, Laird WRE, Lumley PJ. Ultrasound in dentistry. Part 2 – periodontology and endodontics. *J Dent* 1992; 20: 11–7.

Walmsley AD, Laird WRE, Williams AR. A model system to demonstrate the role of cavitational activity in ultrasonic scaling. *J Dent Res* 1984; 63: 1162–5.

Walmsley AD, Laird WRE, Williams AR. Gas bubble fragmentation in an ultrasonic field. *Ultrasonics* 1985; 23: 170–2.

Walmsley AD, Laird WRE, Williams AR. Displacement amplitude as a measure of the acoustic output of ultrasonic scalers. *Dent Mater* 1986; 2: 97–100.

Walmsley AD, Laird WRE, Williams AR. Dental plaque removal by cavitational activity during ultrasonic scaling. *J Clin Periodontol* 1988; 15: 539–43.

Walmsley AD, Lea SC, Felver B, King DC, Price GJ. Mapping cavitation activity around dental ultrasonic tips. *Clin Oral Invest* 2013; 17: 1227–34.

Walmsley AD, Lea SC, Landini G, Moses AJ. Advances in power driven pocket/root instrumentation. *J Clin Periodontol* 2008; 35(Suppl 8): 22–8.

Walmsley AD, Walsh TF, Laird WRE, Williams AR. Effects of cavitational activity on the root surface of teeth during ultrasonic scaling. *J Clin Periodontol* 1990; 17: 306–12.

Walmsley AD, Williams AR. Acoustic absorption within human teeth during ultrasonic descaling. *J Dent* 1986; 14: 2–6.

WHAT IS ULTRASONIC INSTRUMENTATION?

Chapter 4

Ultrasonic tip design and selection

CHAPTER OBJECTIVES

On completion of this chapter, the student will be able to:

1. Identify and define key elements of design common to all ultrasonic tips.

2. Explain the influence of each element of design on the clinical performance of the ultrasonic tip.

3. Recognize variables which influence tip selection.

4. Select a tip design appropriate for the treatment objective and anatomy of the treatment site.

It was explained in Chapter 3 that ultrasonic instruments ablate and disrupt deposits by vibratory and biophysical mechanisms produced by a blunt metal tip oscillating at an ultrasonic frequency (Walmsley et al., 1984; Khambay and Walmsley, 1999), and that these mechanisms of action are influenced by several operational variables, including design of the blunt tip. The design of the tip is also one of several instrumentation technique variables presented in Chapter 6, which influence both deposit removal and root substance loss. Consequently, proper tip selection is a critical step in the implementation of successful debridement instrumentation.

ANATOMY OF AN ULTRASONIC TIP

All ultrasonic tips oscillate in an elliptical pattern, which disperses kinetic energy to each surface of the tip, rendering each surface of the *active* area of the tip clinically useful (Chapter 3). The active area of the tip is the free, unconstrained end of the tip at which displacement amplitude is maximized (see Figure 3.24). It extends approximately 4 mm in length from the last antinode to the terminal end of the tip. During ultrasonic instrumentation, the surfaces within the active area of the tip are adapted to the tooth surface. Figure 4.1 illustrates each surface and the active area of the ultrasonic tip.

The point of the tip, because of its small surface area, exerts a very concentrated output of energy that can easily and significantly damage the root surface. Consequently, the oscillating tip should never be adapted in a manner that places the point of the tip in contact with the root surface. Proper adaptation of the tip is presented in Chapters 6 and 7.

Delivery of cooling water to the tip is either internal (magnetostrictive only) or external (piezoelectric or magnetostrictive) to the tip (Figure 4.2). External delivery may allow the

Ultrasonic Periodontal Debridement: Theory and Technique, First Edition. Marie D. George, Timothy G. Donley and Philip M. Preshaw.
© 2014 John Wiley & Sons, Inc. Published 2014 by John Wiley & Sons, Inc.

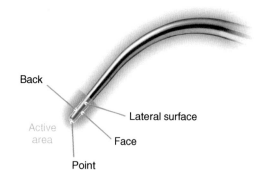

Figure 4.1 The various surfaces of an ultrasonic tip

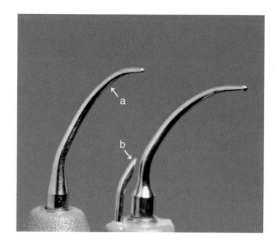

Figure 4.2 Comparison of tips with (a) internal and (b) external water portals

diameter of the tip to be slightly narrower than a comparable tip with internal water delivery. An advantage of internal tubing is that the water is delivered closer in proximity to the active area of the tip. While this more focused delivery probably allows the clinician to better manage the spray of water emitted, it does not reduce the amount of aerosol contamination produced during ultrasonic scaling (Rivera-Hidalgo et al., 1999).

KEY ELEMENTS OF TIP DESIGN

In order to utilize ultrasonic instrumentation as the primary means of periodontal debridement

Table 4.1 Key elements of ultrasonic tip design

Element	Impact
Dimension Diameter (width) of the active area of the tip **Shape** Shape of the active area in cross section	• Degree of force • Amount of cavitation • Degree of contact
Geometry Number of planes crossed by the shank **Profile** Number of bends in tip	• Access to treatment site • Degree of contact

therapy, an adequate variety of tip designs are needed to effectively implement the staged approach to debridement proposed in Chapter 1 and presented in Chapter 6. Accordingly, manufacturers of ultrasonic instruments offer an assortment of tip configurations. Unlike the classification of hand instruments, which is fairly standardized among manufacturers, the systems used by manufacturers to identify and classify ultrasonic tip styles vary greatly, making tip selection and/or comparison by name or color-code complicated. Tip selection is simplified and made more precise by assessing key elements of design that are common to all ultrasonic tips (Table 4.1).

Tip dimension

The dimension, or *diameter*, of the tip is the width or thickness of the tip in the active area. Currently, tips fall into three categories by diameter: standard diameter, slim diameter, and ultraslim diameter (Figure 4.3).

The designation of standard, slim, or ultraslim diameter is an approximation, as standardization of widths (as measured in millimeters) for each category does not exist. Although the specific diameter of the tips in each category may vary

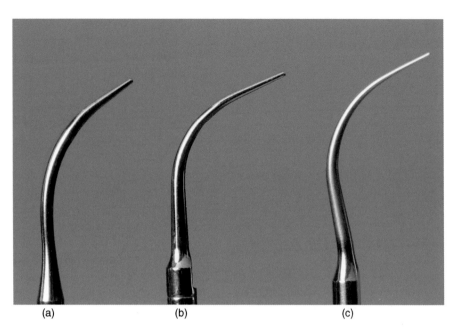

Figure 4.3 Comparison of the various ultrasonic tip diameters. (a) standard diameter; (b) slim diameter; (c) ultraslim diameter

Table 4.2 Classification of ultrasonic tips by diameter

Diameter	Traits
Standard	• Greater mass • Wide, robust diameter • Range from flat and broad to cylindrical in shape • Straight geometry • Also referred to as "traditional" or "scaling" tips
Slim	• Less mass • Reduced in diameter; ~30–40% thinner than standard diameter tips • May be rectangular or cylindrical in shape • Straight or curved geometry • Also known as "thin," "modified," "microultrasonic," or "perio" tips
Ultraslim	• Least mass • Narrowest in diameter; ~40% thinner than slim diameter tips • Cylindrical in shape • Straight geometry • Also known as "extra-thin" tips

slightly among manufacturers, there is within each category some consistency in the physical structure of the tips (Table 4.2).

The diameter of the tip primarily influences both the degree of force exerted and the amount of cavitational and streaming forces produced by the oscillating tip.

Influence of tip diameter on degree of force exerted

As previously explained, the net force exerted by an object (i.e., the oscillating ultrasonic tip) is a product of the object's mass (m) multiplied by its acceleration (Hewitt, 1997) (Figure 4.4).

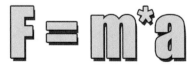

Figure 4.4 Newton's Second Law of Motion. Net force equals mass multiplied by acceleration

The mass of an object is a measure in kilograms (kg) of the amount of matter in the object. Mass and force are directly proportional; therefore more mass equals greater force (Hewitt, 1997).

Given the influence of object mass on force, the mass (indicated by diameter) of the oscillating tip affects the degree of root surface damage and the efficiency of calculus removal, as the two are directly related.

At a given power setting or lateral force, significant increases in root substance loss occur with wide diameter compared with narrow or probe-shaped tips across all parameters of the root surface defect – width, depth, and volume (Jepsen et al., 2004) (Figure 4.5).

The distinction between the depth and volume of the root surface defect is important. Defect depth appears to be a measure of the instrument's capacity for root damage, whereas defect volume may be a gauge for the instrument's efficacy of calculus removal (Flemmig et al., 1998a,b). This means that if the tips are oscillating against calculus, instead of root surface, the wider diameter tips are more efficacious at calculus removal compared to narrow diameter tips.

Influence of tip diameter on cavitation and microstreaming

The dimensions of the tip may be more influential than the displacement amplitude in the generation of cavitation (Walmsley et al., 2013).

At any given displacement amplitude, unloaded wide diameter tips typically produce greater cavitational and streaming forces at the antinodes than unloaded slim diameter tips. This is attributed to the wider dimensions being more capable of displacing larger volumes of water (so producing greater cavitational and microstreaming forces) than narrower dimensions (Khambay and Walmsley, 1999; Felver et al., 2009; Walmsley et al., 2013).

However, the application of load (lateral pressure) increases the amount of cavitational activity occurring at the clinically pertinent active area of slim diameter tips more so than with wide diameter tips (Walmsley et al., 2013).

Influence of tip diameter on access to the treatment site

Slim diameter tips were designed with the intent of improving penetration to the base of the pocket because of their thinner, probe-like diameter. Depth of penetration into the periodontal pocket has been assessed in studies by evidence of instrumentation to the connective tissue attachment (Kawanami et al., 1988; Dragoo et al., 1992) or to the apical plaque border (APB) (Clifford et al., 1999). It can be argued that assessing the APB is a more useful measurement of instrument penetration (Chan et al., 2000), and that penetration past the APB, to the connective tissue attachment, may not be necessary

	Magnetostrictive slim	Piezoelectric slim	Piezoelectric standard	Magnetostrictive standard
Defect width	383.2 (17.3)	582.6 (40.6)	618.09 (9.4)	851.8 (19.6)
Defect depth	7.4 (0.0)	16.2 (0.3)	22.2 (1.0)	55.9 (0.4)
Defect volume	70.8 (0.4)	96.6 (1.6)	254.4 (5.2)	336.8 (11.8)

Figure 4.5 Defect values following three reciprocal (forward and backward) strokes at medium power setting, 0.7 N lateral pressure, and 0° angulation demonstrate an increase in root substance loss occurring with wide diameter compared with slim diameter tips. Data compiled from information found in Jepsen et al., 2004

or desirable (Claffey et al., 1988; Clifford et al., 1999).

Using disruption of the APB as the benchmark, standard and slim diameter tips are comparable (i.e., not statistically different) in their ability to adequately penetrate deep pockets (Kawanami et al., 1988; Dragoo et al., 1992; Clifford et al., 1999). This is noteworthy, as pocket depth is often (but mistakenly) cited by manufacturers and authors as an indication for use of a tip.

However, slim diameter tips do improve access to furcation anatomy and facilitate the effective use of ultrasonic instrumentation for prophylaxis procedures. Ultrasonic debridement with a narrow diameter tip has been demonstrated to be more effective than a standard Gracey curette in decreasing inflammation and motile forms of bacteria in Class II and Class III furcations, most likely due to better access resulting from the narrower diameter of the ultrasonic tip (Leon and Vogel, 1987). In patients with healthier periodontal tissues, the thin diameter of a slim or ultraslim tip facilitates access into the sulcus, expanding the utilization of ultrasonic instruments to prophylaxis procedures (Novaes Junior et al., 2004).

Tip shape

The *shape* of the tip denotes the shape of the active area in cross section, typically designed as either rectangular or circular (Figure 4.6). Tips with a rectangular cross section may be also be described as being "flat and broad" or "curette-like," while tips with a circular cross section are more commonly referred to as being "cylindrical" or "probe-like." Keep in mind that the shape of the tip is independent of the diameter of the tip: there are tips in the slim diameter category with a rectangular cross section, just as there are tips in the standard diameter category with a cylindrical cross section.

Similar to the impact of diameter, tip shape contributes to the degree of force exerted and the amount of cavitation produced by the oscillating tip. The surfaces of a rectangular shaped tip meet to form an edge. This edge, like the point of the tip, exerts a concentrated output of energy because of its reduced surface area, which may be beneficial for the scaling of heavy and/or tenacious calculus, but is detrimental for debridement of the root surface (Jepsen et al., 2004; Lea et al., 2009). Lea et al. found almost no difference in the depth and volume of root surface defects produced by slim diameter rectangular and cylindrical tips even though the cylindrical tip was oscillating at a higher displacement amplitude, demonstrating the greater force exerted by the rectangular tip. A rectangular shaped tip also produces more cavitation than a cylindrical tip of equal diameter, as its paddle-like shape is more conducive to the displacement of water (Khambay and Walmsley, 1999; Felver et al., 2009).

The shape of the tip additionally and notably influences the degree of contact achieved between the tip and the surface to be treated. As the primary mechanism of debridement is mechanical (Chapter 3), success is contingent on contact of the active area of the tip to the treatment surface; the greater the degree of contact between the active tip and the treatment surface, the greater the likelihood for thorough disruption and removal of the deposits.

A greater degree of contact results when the shape of the active portion of the tip conforms to the anatomy of the treatment site. For example, consider how the convex back surface of the cylindrical tip in Figure 4.6 better conforms to a root surface concavity than the relatively straight back surface of the rectangular tip.

Tip geometry

The *geometry* of the tip is defined by the number of planes that the shank of the tip crosses. The majority of tip designs extend in only one plane and so are geometrically *straight*. Tips which are *curved* in geometry are semi-spiral in design with a curvature to the side that extends the tip into a second plane (Figure 4.7).

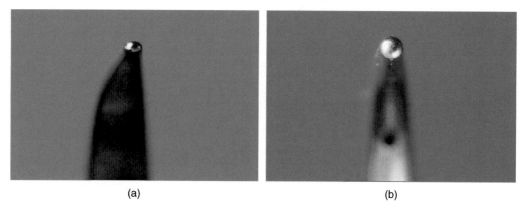

(a)   (b)

Figure 4.6 The shape of an ultrasonic tip in cross-section may be (a) rectangular or (b) circular

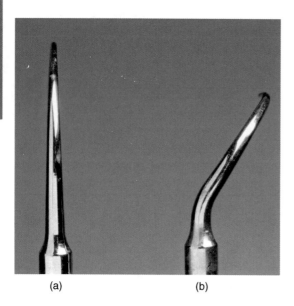

(a)   (b)

Figure 4.7 The geometry of an ultrasonic tip may be (a) straight or (b) curved

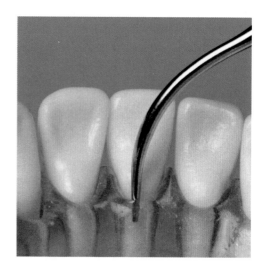

Figure 4.8 A straight ultrasonic tip readily adapts to the characteristically flat root surfaces of anterior teeth

The geometry of the tip affects the clinician's ability to access the treatment site and make adequate contact with the surface to be treated.

Influence of tip geometry on access to the treatment site

A straight shank is appropriate when access to the treatment site is uncomplicated, such as with the coronal surfaces of all teeth and the typically flat root surfaces of anterior teeth (Figure 4.8). The straight alignment also allows the clinician to easily estimate the position of the tip within the periodontal pocket (Clifford et al., 1999).

When access to the treatment site is complex, as generally occurs when instrumenting the root surfaces of posterior teeth, a curved shank is indicated. The contra-angle of the shank is required to adapt the tip around the maximal contour of the tooth surface so that the tip reaches the site and is in a position that facilitates proper ultrasonic instrumentation technique (Chapter 6) (Figure 4.9).

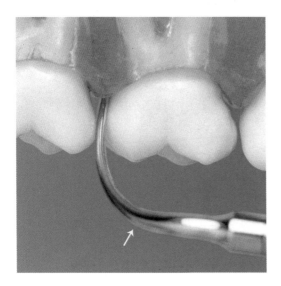

Figure 4.9 The contra-angle (indicated by arrow) of a curved tip facilitates access and adaptation of the active tip area to posterior root surfaces

Influence of tip geometry on degree of contact

Subsequent to accessing the treatment site, the tip then needs to make adequate contact with deposits in order for disruption and removal to occur. The geometry of the tip influences the degree of contact achieved in that a tip with a straight shank typically is straight in the active area as well, whereas a tip with a curved shank may arc in the active area (Figure 4.10).

A straight active tip area conforms to the curvatures of the tooth to a lesser degree than does a curved active tip area (Figure 4.11). This lesser degree of contact is not necessarily inadequate, as the disruption of calculus and biofilm require different degrees of contact. During the scaling of moderate amounts of calculus, a lesser degree of contact is sufficient for the tip to adequately engage and break the mass of calculus; in fact, the majority of standard diameter tips are straight in alignment.

In contrast, a greater degree of contact is required for the tip to predictably engage and disrupt biofilm and light calculus; accordingly, slim diameter tips are designed with both straight and curved geometry.

Tip profile

The profile of the tip refers to the number of bends placed in the shank of a straight tip to

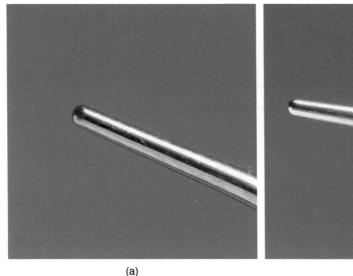
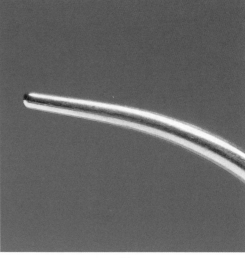

(a)   (b)

Figure 4.10 Comparison of the active areas of a (a) straight and (b) curved ultrasonic tip

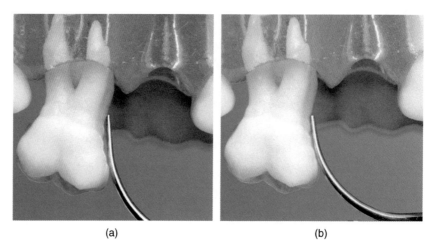

(a)   (b)

Figure 4.11 The degree of conformity to the mesial concavity of a maxillary molar achieved by (a) a straight tip compared to (b) a curved tip. Note that the gap, visible between the straight tip and the concavity, is closed by adaptation of the curved tip

facilitate access. Most common are straight tip designs with a single bend; tips designed with a double or triple bend are also available for improved adaptation around line angles and into interproximal spaces (Figure 4.12).

Several manufacturers commonly identify magnetostrictive straight tips with a single bend as the #10 design, a double bend as #100, and a triple bend as #1000, but, as previously mentioned, these labels are neither

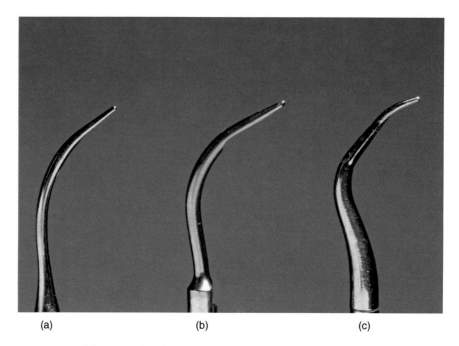

(a)   (b)   (c)

Figure 4.12 Comparison of the various bends placed in the shank of a straight ultrasonic tip. (a) single bend; (b) double bend; (c) triple bend

standardized nor universal among generator types (magnetostrictive and piezoelectric) or manufacturers. However, there is one designation that a majority of manufacturers do utilize that warrants discussion, as its use can be misleading and confusing to the clinician implementing two-stage debridement instrumentation. This discussion of the use of the label "universal" as it relates to tip design is presented in Box 4.1.

Box 4.1: "Universal" tip design: A misused label

Ultrasonic tips designated as *"universal"* in design are common among manufacturers. This is a concern, as the label is ambiguous and does not align with the contemporary staged approach to debridement instrumentation.

A quick search of the term "universal" on www.merriam-webster.com produces definitions such as "including without limit or exception," "operative everywhere or under all conditions," and "adjustable to meet varied requirements." Hence, labeling a tip as "universal" infers that it can be effectively adapted to the contours of any surface and accomplish both thorough scaling of calculus and debridement of biofilm without over-instrumentation of the root surface.

Tips labeled as "universal" are characteristically straight with one bend (aka #10), but may be cylindrical or rectangular in cross-section, standard or slim diameter, with an indication for use for either scaling or debridement. Given how diameter, shape, and alignment influence the performance of the tip, the range of configurations available with definitive indications for use contradicts the definition of "universal."

The fact remains that an adequate variety of tip designs are necessary to accomplish the objectives of periodontal debridement therapy. A truly "universal" tip design is a fallacy and the use of the label "universal" by manufacturers, clinicians, authors, and faculty is strongly discouraged.

As the number of bends in the shank increases, the length of the terminal portion of the tip decreases. The length of either a single-bend or double bend tip allows for sufficient penetration to the base of a deep pocket; but the length of a triple-bend tip is reduced by that third bend in the shank, limiting utilization to shallow pockets and supragingival surfaces.

Table 4.3 summarizes the influence of each element of design to the clinical performance of a tip.

TIP SELECTION

With the understanding of how these key elements of design influence tip performance, accurate tip selection is expedited. As the primary variables to consider when selecting a tip are (i) the type of deposit to be removed and (ii) the anatomy of the surface to be treated, assessment of the treatment site and knowledge of root surface morphology are essential. Figure 4.13 illustrates these variables as a decision tree for proper tip selection.

Tip selection decision #1: Type of deposit

The type of deposit presenting at the treatment site determines how much force is needed from the tip for efficient removal (Figure 4.14). As previously established, the force exerted by the tip increases as both mass (diameter) of the tip and displacement amplitude (power setting) increase. Calculus removal requires a higher degree of force than does the disruption of biofilm. Therefore, if moderate amounts of calculus predominate the treatment site, a standard diameter tip (operated at higher displacement amplitude) is indicated to produce the greater force required to efficiently remove/reduce the calculus deposits. When biofilm and light calculus prevail, a slim diameter tip (oscillating at a reduced displacement) produces a lesser degree of force appropriate for definitive debridement of these types of deposits without over-instrumentation of the root surface.

ULTRASONIC TIP DESIGN AND SELECTION

Table 4.3 Influence of elements of tip design to tip performance

Variable		Force (F)	Cavitation (CA) and Microstreaming (AMS)	Access	Degree of Contact
Tip diameter	Standard	↑ F	↑ CA/AMS at anti-node	Adequate penetration of pocket	
	Slim	↓ F	↑ CA/AMS at active area		
Tip shape	Rectangular	↑ F	↑ CA/AMS		Adequate for calculus removal
	Cylindrical	↓ F	↓ CA/AMS		↑ conformity for biofilm disruption
Tip geometry	Straight			Adequate to coronal surfaces and anterior roots	Adequate for calculus removal
	Curved			↑ access to posterior root surfaces	↑ conformity for biofilm disruption
Tip profile	1–2 bends			↑ access to base of pocket	
	3 bends			↑ access to IP space	

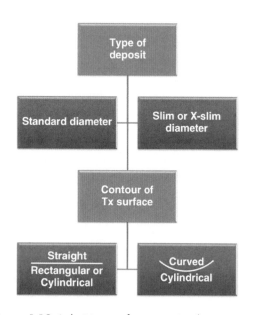

Figure 4.13 A decision tree for proper tip selection

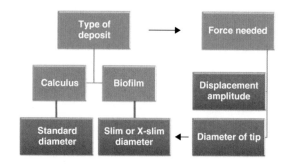

Figure 4.14 Process followed to select the appropriate tip diameter

Tip selection decision #2: Contour of the treatment site

Once the proper diameter of the tip is determined, the contour assessed at the treatment site predicates the shape and geometry of the tip that will provide the preferred degree of

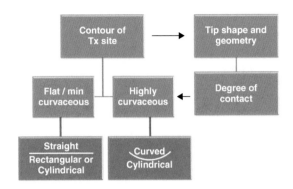

Figure 4.15 Process followed to select the appropriate tip shape

contact (Figure 4.15). Both elements – shape and geometry – must be taken into consideration with the type of deposit to be removed.

When the contour of the treatment site is minimally curvaceous or flat, as typical of most coronal surfaces and the roots of the anterior teeth, either a rectangular or cylindrical straight tip will provide an effective degree of contact for the scaling of calculus. Recall that a rectangular shaped tip is more aggressive than a cylindrical tip of the same diameter, making it more efficient at breaking calculus, but also more damaging to root surfaces (Jepsen et al., 2004; Lea et al., 2009). And so, for the debridement of biofilm on the root surfaces of anterior teeth, only a cylindrically shaped tip (straight or curved) should be used.

Where tooth contours are more curvaceous (posterior root surfaces), cylindrical or rectangular straight tips can adequately engage to fracture/reduce a mass of calculus (remember all standard tips are straight). However, only a cylindrical curved tip *with the arc extending into the active area* can predictably engage biofilm in highly curved areas. (See Figure 4.10.) This is an important distinction to make, as not all curved tips continue to arc into the active area, a difference which is clinically significant (Figure 4.16).

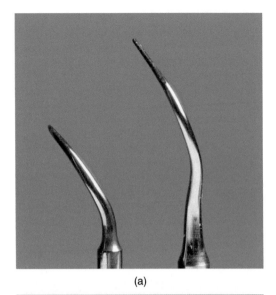

(a)

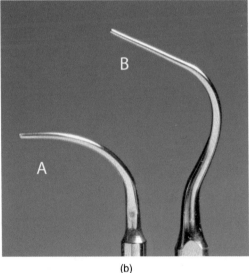

(b)

Figure 4.16 Comparison of the active areas of different curved tips. (a) While both tips are categorized as "curved" tips because of the contra-angle in the shank, (b) the arced active area of tip A will better conform to highly curved areas than the straight active area of tip B

The labeling of the tip as "curved" is indicative of the contra-angle in the shank, not the geometry of the active area.

Box 4.2: But what about pocket depth?

Pocket depth is often, and mistakenly, cited by manufacturers and authors as an indication for use of a tip. Citing a range of pocket depths (≤4 mm or >4 mm) as an indication for use is not supported by the evidence, but more importantly, is invalidated by the studies that demonstrate adequate and comparable penetration of deep pockets by both standard and slim diameter tips.

As just discussed, the criteria for tip utilization are type of deposit and anatomy of the treatment site. As only a few select tip designs are limited to use in shallow pockets (triple bend because of short length) or supragingival surfaces (beavertail), the use of pocket depth as a criterion for tip selection should be avoided.

Table 4.4 summarizes the process of tip selection.

TIP UTILIZATION

In Chapter 6, it will be explained that the principles of ultrasonic instrumentation technique are applicable to all tip designs; that is to say that,

while the design of the tip will change according to the type of deposit and contour of the site, the instrumentation technique used with each tip will not change. That said, a few tip designs with unique features warrant further discussion to optimize utilization.

Curved tips

To accomplish proper debridement of the full circumference of posterior root surfaces, a complementary pair of area-specific curved tips is necessary. The contra-angles of each tip in the pair curve in opposite directions, with the spiral of one tip arced to the left and the spiral of the other tip arced to the right, hence the generic labels "left curved tip" and "right curved tip" (Figure 4.17).

Each tip is designed to optimize instrumentation in specific areas of the dentition (i.e., each tip is area specific). Areas of utilization are designated by the ability to achieve vertical adaptation with the point of the tip directed away from the tooth (Figure 4.18). This approach takes full advantage of the curvature of the tip, optimizing conformity to the contours of the surface while preventing the point from damaging the root surface.

Table 4.4 Tip selection guide

Type of deposit	Tooth surface contour	Tip diameter	Tip shape	Tip geometry	Tip profile
Moderate calculus	Flat or Curvaceous All coronal surfaces All root surfaces	Standard	Cylindrical or Rectangular	Straight	1–3 bends
Biofilm/ slight calculus	Flat or Minimally Curvaceous All coronal surfaces Anterior root surfaces	Slim or Ultraslim	Cylindrical Rectangular (coronal surfaces only)	Straight or Curved	1 or 2 bends Triple bend (coronal surfaces only due to rectangular shape)
	Highly Curvaceous Posterior root surfaces	Slim	Cylindrical	Curved	Not applicable to curved tips

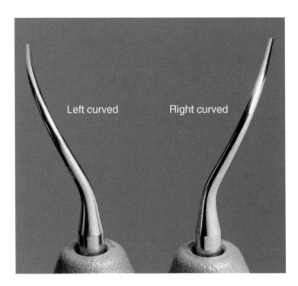

Figure 4.17 Left and right curved tips as viewed from the back of the tips with the point of the tips directed away

Table 4.5 Left and right curved tip utilization guide

Sextant	Right	Anterior	Left
Maxillary arch			
Buccal/facial	LEFT curved	RIGHT curved	RIGHT curved
Palatal	RIGHT curved	LEFT curved	LEFT curved
Mandibular arch			
Lingual	LEFT curved	RIGHT curved	RIGHT curved
Buccal/facial	RIGHT curved	LEFT curved	LEFT curved

Accordingly, the left curved tip is utilized in the maxillary arch in the right buccal and left palatal sextants, and in the mandibular arch in the left buccal and right lingual sextants. The right curved tip properly adapts to the maxillary right palatal and left buccal sextants, and the mandibular left lingual and right buccal sextants.

Although the curved tips are predominantly utilized to debride posterior teeth, they can be effectively adapted to the anterior teeth as well, replacing the use of a straight slim tip (Figure 4.19). Table 4.5 summarizes the designated areas of utilization for each of the curved tips.

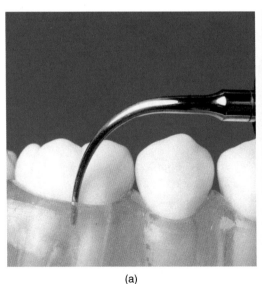

(a)

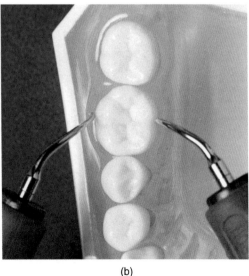

(b)

Figure 4.18 Vertical adaptation of curved tips to #30 (FDI 46). (a) adaptation of the right curved tip as viewed from the buccal perspective; (b) occlusal view illustrating that, when correctly adapted, the contra-angle of the right tip curves toward the buccal surface, with the contra-angle of the left tip curving toward the lingual surface

ULTRASONIC TIP DESIGN AND SELECTION

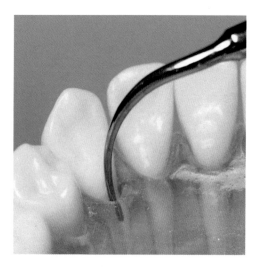

Figure 4.19 Utilization of a right curved tip in the mandibular anterior lingual sextant

Furcation ball tips

Adequate debridement of furcation surfaces is challenging because of the posterior location of the multi-rooted teeth and the concave or irregularly contoured anatomy (Takacs et al.,

1993). To be expected, the highest levels of residual deposits in furcations are found on the surfaces most difficult to access: internally on the domes of both maxillary and mandibular furcas, and externally at the mesial entrance of maxillary furcations and the buccal entrance of mandibular furcations (Takacs et al., 1993). Consequently, effective debridement of a furcational defect is highly dependent on the shape and dimension of the instrument tip.

Modified forms of the left and right curved tips are indicated specifically for the debridement of furcations. At the terminal end of the spiral shank is a sphere with a diameter of 0.8 mm, designed to improve contact with the predominantly concave contours of furcations without the risk of root gouging by a pointed tip (Figure 4.20).

Use of the left/right ball-end tips results in more effective deposit removal in both maxillary and mandibular furcations than slim curved ultrasonic tips (Takacs et al., 1993) and Gracey curettes (Oda and Ishikawa, 1989). This greater effectiveness is most likely attributable to the superior accessibility to the furcational surfaces and improved conformity to the anatomy

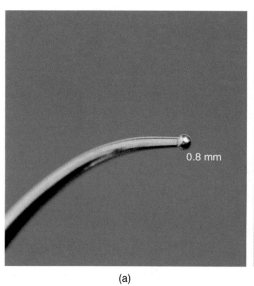

(a)

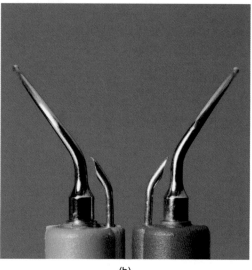

(b)

Figure 4.20 Furcation-specific, ball-end tips are designed with (a) a sphere at the terminal end of either straight or (b) left and right curved shanks

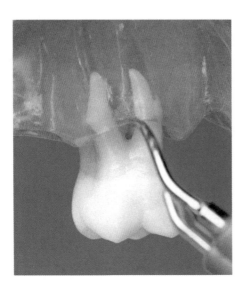

Figure 4.21 Adaptation of a ball-end tip in the furcation mimics that of a Nabers furcation probe

Table 4.6 Left and right furcation ball tip utilization guide

Sextant	Right	Left
Maxillary arch		
Buccal	RIGHT Ball	LEFT Ball
Palatal	LEFT Ball	RIGHT Ball
Mandibular arch		
Lingual	RIGHT Ball	LEFT Ball
Buccal	LEFT Ball	RIGHT Ball

afforded by a spherically shaped tip (Takacs et al., 1993). Superior access is gained because the ball-end tip can be adapted within the furcation like a Nabers (furcation) probe, without risk of root gouging (Figure 4.21).

Similar to the pointed left/right curved tips, the left/right ball-end tips are area-specific, but with the sextant designation being the opposite of that of the curved tips due to the different method of adaptation used (like a Nabers probe). Table 4.6 designates the areas of utilization for the left and right furcation ball tips.

Implant tips

As the titanium surfaces of dental implants that are exposed to the oral cavity can be altered by metal tips (Thomson-Neal et al., 1989; Rapley et al., 1990; Augthun et al., 1998; Bailey et al., 1998; Park et al., 2012; Mann et al., 2012), a variety of non-metal ultrasonic tips have been developed (Figure 4.22). These tips, made of carbon fiber or plastic, are suitable to debride smooth titanium surfaces without alteration (Sato et al., 2004; Kawashima et al., 2007), but can cause significant surface disruption of

both plasma and hydroxyapatite coated surfaces (Thomson-Neal et al., 1989; Augthun et al., 1998; Bailey et al., 1998; Ramaglia et al., 2006). Additionally, the diameter of these tips tends to be bulky, which compromises access, and consequently, effectiveness. The effectiveness of various methods of instrumentation in debriding dental implants is addressed in Chapter 2.

Considering the safe use of these plastic and carbon tips on titanium, expanding utilization to the debridement of restoration margins seems appropriate, although at the time of this writing, no evidence either supporting or contradicting such an indication has been published.

Diamond-coated tips

Ultrasonic tips coated with fine or medium grit diamonds are indicated for use only under direct vision during open flap debridement (Figure 4.23).

The diamond coating provides multiple cutting edges to facilitate substantially faster calculus removal compared to regular ultrasonic tips (Yukna et al., 1997; Scott et al., 1999; Yukna et al., 2007). As efficiency of calculus removal and root substance loss are directly related, diamond-coated tips also result in significantly greater root surface removal and roughness than similarly shaped regular ultrasonic tips (Lavespere et al., 1996; Yukna et al., 1997; Vastardis et al., 2005). See Figure 4.24.

ULTRASONIC TIP DESIGN AND SELECTION

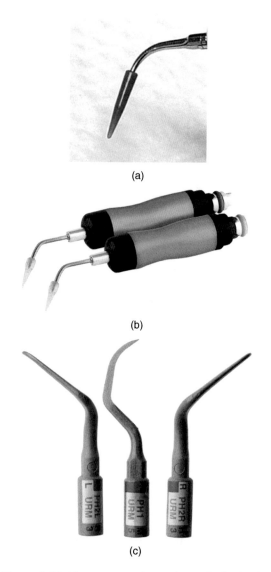

(a)

(b)

(c)

Figure 4.22 Ultrasonic tips designed specifically for the safe debridement of dental implants include (a, b) plastic-covered tips and (c) tips made of carbon fiber. Images (a) Cavitron SofTip™ (b) GentleCLEAN™ magnetostrictive (courtesy of Parkell, Inc.) and (c) Satelec piezo tips (courtesy of ACTEON North America)

Because of the substantial amount of root surface removed within a very short application time, diamond-coated ultrasonic tips should be used with caution and only during periodontal surgery in areas that will be covered with gingiva after healing (Lavespere et al., 1996; Vastardis et al., 2005; Yukna et al., 2007).

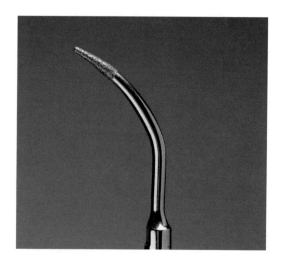

Figure 4.23 Diamond-coated ultrasonic tip

EFFECT OF WEAR ON TIP PERFORMANCE

To review, the mechanical and biophysical mechanisms of ultrasonic debridement are influenced by the displacement amplitude of the oscillating tip (Chapter 3), with the area of maximum displacement amplitude (the active area) being approximately 4 mm in length from the last anti-node to the point of the tip.

With routine clinical usage, the ultrasonic tip may wear and become reduced in length. This reduction in length occurs in the active area of the tip, consequently reducing the displacement amplitude (Figure 4.25) and ultimately affecting the clinical performance of the tip (Lea et al., 2006).

The bar graph in Figure 4.25 illustrates that for a slim diameter tip oscillating at a medium power setting with 0.5 N lateral pressure (red bar), the displacement amplitude is reduced with 1 mm of wear by a mean of 50%, from approximately 22 μm when unworn to 11 μm, with greater lateral pressure (green bar) reducing the displacement amplitude even further. Increasing the power setting of a worn tip in an attempt to compensate for the reduction in performance

	10 strokes	20 strokes	30 strokes	Per stroke
Diamond US tip	46.2 (18.4)	95.4 (28.3)	142.0 (42.3)	4.7
Regular US tip	10.7* (6.5)	18.2* (8.7)	21.6* (27.1)	0.9
Gracey curette	15.0* (14.8)	25.7* (15.5)	33.2* (24.6)	1.3

* Significantly different from diamond-coated tip

Figure 4.24 Root defect depth following 10, 20, and 30 strokes. Ultrasonic tips were operated at medium power setting, 1N lateral pressure, unspecified angulation. (Data compiled from information found in Vastardis et al., 2005)

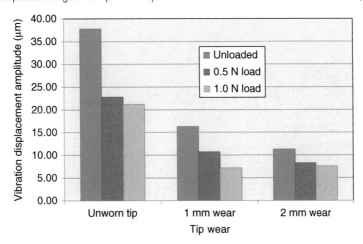

Figure 4.25 Graph demonstrating the effect of wear on ultrasonic tip vibration displacement amplitude of a slim diameter straight cylindrical tip under loaded and unloaded conditions. (*Source*: Lea et al., 2006. Modified with permission of John Wiley & Sons.)

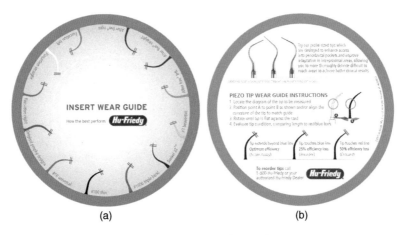

(a)   (b)

Figure 4.26 Wear guides for (a) magnetostrictive and (b) piezoelectric ultrasonic tips. Images courtesy of Hu-Friedy Mfg Co., LLC, Chicago IL, USA.

Table 4.7 Authors' recommendations for basic (minimum) tip setup

Tip Design	Indication for Use	Rationale for Inclusion
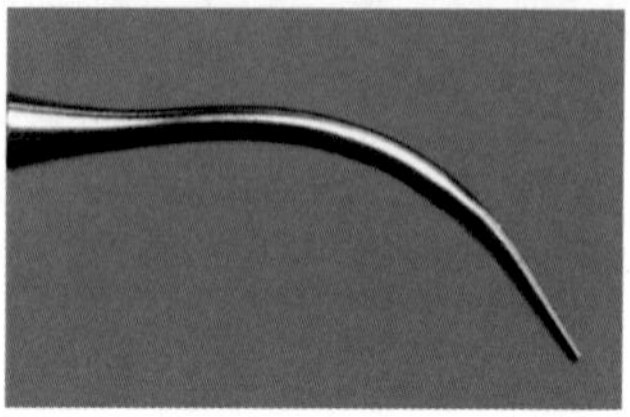 **Figure 4.27** Standard 1-bend	Removal/reduction of moderate-heavy calculus	The longer length of a tip with 1-bend ensures adequate penetration to the base of the pocket
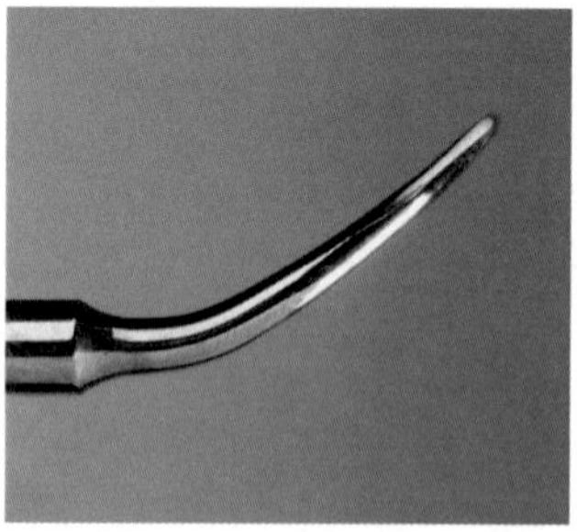 **Figure 4.28** Slim Left curved 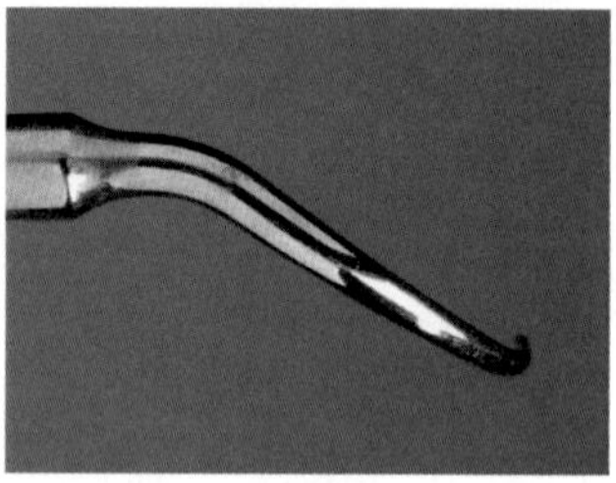 **Figure 4.29** Slim Right curved	Definitive debridement of biofilm and light calculus	Ensures adequate adaptation to highly curvaceous tooth contours AND to less curvaceous/flat contours, negating the need for a slim straight tip
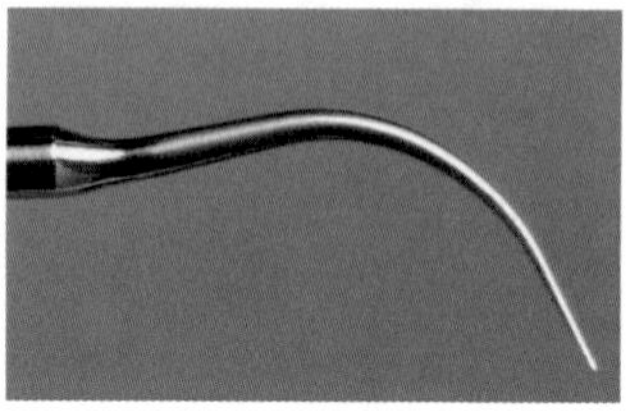 **Figure 4.30** Ultraslim	Definitive debridement of biofilm and light calculus	Facilitates access to areas where even slim diameter is too broad, such as tight contacts and areas with healthier or tight tissue tone

resulting from wear is ineffective and thus not recommended (Lea et al., 2006).

Tip wear must, therefore, be monitored regularly to ensure adequate clinical performance and to identify tips that should be discarded due to wear. Wear guides, designed for easy assessment of tip length, are brand-specific and provided by each manufacturer of ultrasonic tips (Figure 4.26). However, manufacturers typically recommend replacing the tip when 2 mm, or 50%, of the active area is lost, whereas the significant reduction in displacement amplitude after 1 mm of wear observed by Lea et al. may warrant the earlier replacement of slim diameter tips.

BASIC TIP SETUP

With such an abundant assortment of tips available in the market, determining which tip designs are essential to include in the instrument set can be puzzling. It is the opinion of these authors that, at the minimum, four tip designs should be available to predictably carry out thorough debridement of variable deposits from the different site morphologies encountered during any nonsurgical periodontal procedure – initial therapy, periodontal maintenance, or prophylaxis. The minimal or basic ultrasonic tip setup suggested by these authors is offered in Table 4.7.

REFERENCES

Augthun M, Tinschert J, Huber A. In vitro studies on the effect of cleaning methods on different implant surfaces. *J Periodontol* 1998; 69: 857–64.

Bailey GM, Gardner JS, Day MK, Kovanda BJ. Implant surface alterations from a nonmetallic ultrasonic tip. *J West Soc Periodontal Abstr* 1998; 46: 69–73.

Chan YK, Needleman IG, Clifford LR. Comparison of four methods of assessing root surface debridement. *J Periodontol* 2000; 71: 385–93.

Claffey N, Loos B, Gantes B, Martin M, Heins P, Egelberg J. The relative effects of therapy and

periodontal disease on loss of probing attachment after root debridement. *J Clin Periodontol* 1988; 15: 163–9.

Clifford LR, Needleman IG, Chan YK. Comparison of periodontal pocket penetration by conventional and microultrasonic inserts. *J Clin Periodontol* 1999; 26: 124–30.

Dragoo MR. A clinical evaluation of hand ultrasonic instruments on subgingival debridement. Part I. With unmodified and modified ultrasonic inserts. *Int J Periodontics Restorative Dent* 1992; 12: 310–23.

Felver B, King DC, Lea SC, Price GJ, Walmsley AD. Cavitation occurrence around ultrasonic dental scalers. *Ultrason Sonochem* 2009; 16: 692–7.

Flemmig TF, Petersilka GJ, Mehl A, Hickel R, Klaiber B. The effect of working parameters on root substance removal using a piezoelectric ultrasonic scaler in vitro. *J Clin Periodontol* 1998a; 25: 158–63.

Flemmig TF, Petersilka GJ, Mehl A, Hickel R, Klaiber B. Working parameters of a magnetostrictive ultrasonic scaler influencing root substance removal in vitro. *J Periodontol* 1998b; 69: 547–53.

Hewitt PG, (1997) *Conceptual physics.* 3rd edn. Addison-Wesley Publishing Company, Boston.

Jepsen S, Ayna M, Hedderich J, Eberhard J. Significant influence of scaler tip design on root substance loss resulting from ultrasonic scaling: a laserprofilometric in vitro study. *J Clin Periodontol* 2004; 31: 1003–6.

Kawanami M, Sugaya T, Kato S, Iinuma K, Tate T, Hannan MA et al., Efficacy of an ultrasonic scaler with a periodontal probe-type tip in deep periodontal pockets. *Adv Dent Res* 1988; 2: 405–10.

Kawashima H, Sato S, Kishida M, Yagi H, Matsumoto K, Ito K. Treatment of titanium dental implants with three piezoelectric ultrasonic scalers: an in vivo study. *J Periodontal* 2007; 78: 1689–94.

Khambay BS, Walmsley AD. Acoustic microstreaming detection and measurement around ultrasonic scalers. *J Periodontol* 1999; 70: 626–31.

Lavespere JE, Yukna RA, Rice DA, LeBlanc DM. Root surface removal with diamond-coated ultrasonic instruments: an in vitro and SEM study. *J Periodontol* 1996; 67: 1281–7.

Lea SC, Felver B, Landini G, Walmsley AD. Ultrasonic scaler oscillations and tooth-surface defects. *J Dent Res* 2009; 88: 229–34.

Lea SC, Landini G, Walmsley AD. The effect of wear on ultrasonic scaler tip displacement amplitude. *J Clin Periodontol* 2006; 33: 37–41.

Leon LE, Vogel RI. A comparison of the effectiveness of hand scaling and ultrasonic debridement in furcations as evaluated by differential dark-field microscopy. *J Periodontol* 1987; 58: 86–94.

Mann M, Parmar D, Walmsley AD, Lea SC. Effect of plastic covered ultrasonic scalers on titanium implant surfaces. *Clin Oral Impl Res* 2012; 23: 76–82.

Novaes Junior AB, de Souza SL, Taba M Jr, Grisi MF, Suzigan LC, Tunes RS. Control of gingival inflammation in a teenager population using ultrasonic prophylaxis. *Braz Dent J* 2004; 15: 41–5.

Oda S, Ishikawa I. In vitro effectiveness of a newly-designed ultrasonic scaler tip for furcation areas. *J Periodontol* 1989; 60: 634–9.

Park JB, Jang YJ, Koh M, Choi BK, Kim KK, Ko Y. In vitro analysis of the efficacy of ultrasonic scalers and a toothbrush for removing bacteria from RBM titanium discs. *J Periodontol* 2013; 84: 1191–8.

Ramaglia L, di Lauro AE, Morgese F, Squillace A. Profilometric and standard error of the mean analysis of rough implant surfaces treated with different instrumentations. *Implant Dent* 2006; 15: 77–82.

Rapley JW, Swan RH, Hallmon WW, Mills MP. The surface characteristics produced by various oral hygiene instruments and materials on titanium implant abutments. *Int J Oral Maxillofacial Implants* 1990; 5: 47–52.

Rivera-Hildalgo F, Barnes JB, Harrel SK. Aerosol and splatter production by focused spray and standard ultrasonic inserts. *J Periodontol* 1999; 70: 473–7.

Sato S, Kishida M, Ito K. The comparative effect of ultrasonic scalers on titanium surfaces: an in vitro study. *J Periodontol* 2004; 75: 1269–73.

Scott JB, Steed-Veilands AM, Yukna RA. Improved efficacy of calculus removal in furcations using ultrasonic diamond-coated inserts. *Int J Periodontics Restorative Dent* 1999; 19: 355–61.

Takacs VJ, Lie T, Perala DG, Adams DF. Efficacy of 5 machining instruments in scaling of molar furcations. *J Periodontol* 1993; 64: 228–36.

Thomson-Neal D, Evans GH, Meffert RM. Effects of various prophylactic treatments on titanium, sapphire, and hydroxyapatite-coated implants: an SEM study. *Int J Periodontics Restorative Dent* 1989; 9: 300–11.

Vastardis S, Yukna RA, Rice DA, Mercante D. Root surface removal and resultant surface texture with diamond-coated ultrasonic inserts: an in vitro and SEM study. *J Clin Periodontol* 2005; 32: 467–73.

Walmsley AD, Laird WRE, Williams AR. A model system to demonstrate the role of cavitational activity in ultrasonic scaling. *J Dent Res* 1984; 63: 1162–5.

Walmsley AD, Lea SC, Felver B, King DC, Price GJ. Mapping cavitation activity around dental ultrasonic tips. *Clin Oral Invest* 2013; 17: 1227–34.

Yukna RA, Scott JB, Aichelmann-Reidy ME, LeBlanc DM, Mayer ET. Clinical evaluation of the speed and effectiveness of subgingival calculus removal on single-rooted teeth with diamond-coated ultrasonic tips. *J Periodontol* 1997; 68: 436–42.

Yukna RA, Vastardis S, Mayer ET. Calculus removal with diamond-coated ultrasonic insert in vitro. *J Periodontol* 2007; 78: 122–6.

ULTRASONIC TIP DESIGN AND SELECTION

SECTION III

CLINICAL APPLICATION

Chapter 5

Patient assessment

CHAPTER OBJECTIVES

1. To consider the key aspects of the medical and dental history that are relevant to the management of periodontitis.
2. To describe the clinical factors to assess when deciding which sites require periodontal treatment.
3. To review the parameters to be assessed at diseased sites that will influence decisions about how to treat each site.
4. To consider the medical factors (and other patient factors) that are relevant when planning periodontal therapy.

A detailed and thorough examination of the periodontal tissues is essential to ascertain disease extent (i.e., the distribution of pockets) and severity (i.e., the depth of pockets) in patients with periodontitis. This is routinely achieved by undertaking a full probing chart, recording probing depths at 6 points per tooth throughout the entire dentition. There is no shortcut available for this procedure, and it must be explained to the patient that detailed charting is essential to assess the baseline periodontal status (and therefore inform the diagnosis), to help plan the treatment (i.e., to decide which sites require instrumentation), and to be used as a reference point for assessing the response to the treatment. Measurement of probing depths is a fundamental component of periodontal therapy and decisions about instrumentation are made based on the depth of pockets, along with other factors such as bleeding on probing (BOP), the presence of biofilm and calculus, and other signs of inflammation.

THE PERIODONTAL EXAMINATION

First: listen

The periodontal examination starts with a conversation: why has the patient come to see you, what are their problems, what do they hope to achieve from treatment? It is best to ask open-ended questions that invite the patient to describe, in their own words, what their primary concerns are. Some of the typical sorts of questions that are useful to ask are shown in Box 5.1. As an example, a common complaint from patients with advanced periodontitis is drifting or over-eruption of teeth, resulting in a cosmetic problem (Figure 5.1). It is important to be aware of factors like this from the outset, so that the patient's expectations can be managed: as a clinician, you may be very happy with a generalized reduction in probing depths

Ultrasonic Periodontal Debridement: Theory and Technique, First Edition. Marie D. George, Timothy G. Donley and Philip M. Preshaw.
© 2014 John Wiley & Sons, Inc. Published 2014 by John Wiley & Sons, Inc.

Box 5.1: Useful questions to ask a new patient regarding their periodontal status

You've come to see me regarding your gum health: what sorts of problems have you been experiencing?

Patients may describe a variety of problems: difficulty with chewing certain types of foods, altered speech, difficulty wearing dentures, bleeding gums, concerns about mobile teeth, compromised aesthetics. Alternatively, they may not have any particular symptoms or concerns at all, other than knowing that they have a problem with their gums.

Have you noticed any bleeding from the gums, for example when brushing your teeth, on waking up, or when eating?

Have you noticed if any of your teeth are loose?

Have you had any pain or sensitivity from any of your teeth?

Have you had any treatment for gum problems before?

If the patient has had treatment, ask further questions: when was the treatment done, how many appointments, how long did the treatment visits last for?

Do you smoke?

If the answer is yes, ask further questions: for how many years have they smoked, and how many cigarettes per day? If the patient is an ex-smoker, ask how many years they smoked for, how many cigarettes per day, and also, when did they quit?

Have you had any bad taste or bad breath? Have you noticed any gum swelling?

What do you use for cleaning your teeth?

Find out whether the patient uses a manual or powered brush, or any other cleaning aids such as floss or interproximal brushes. How often do they use them, for example, daily? How long do they spend on their oral hygiene procedures?

What is your understanding of what has caused your gum problems?

This is a really useful question to ask, as it will provide good information regarding the patient's knowledge of the causes of periodontal problems, and will help you frame the discussions about periodontal disease and treatment in terms that are meaningful to the patient.

What would be your ideal outcome following treatment?

This will be linked to their primary complaints. For example, improved aesthetics may be the desired outcome, or eradication of bad breath, or reduced bleeding. It is important to manage the patient's expectations, and to be very honest about what can realistically be achieved as a result of the periodontal therapy. If the nonsurgical periodontal therapy is the first part of a complex treatment approach that might involve, for example, fixed or removable prosthodontics, or orthodontics, or periodontal surgery, it is important that the patient is aware that the appropriateness of performing such complex procedures may well depend on the outcomes of the initial periodontal therapy, the response to treatment, and their ability to maintain a high standard of plaque control.

following treatment, but if the over-erupted tooth is still in the same place following treatment, the patient may not be as pleased! It is essential, therefore, to understand the patient's main concerns so that you can discuss the aims of the treatment with them, and ensure that they are aware of the expected outcomes of your care.

Medical and dental history

Following on from the initial conversation with the patient, and before commencing the clinical examination, a full medical history should be recorded. A systematic approach should always be followed when recording the medical history; health history forms that are completed by the patient and then reviewed by the clinician together with the patient are useful to ensure that nothing is missed (Figure 5.2). Aspects of the

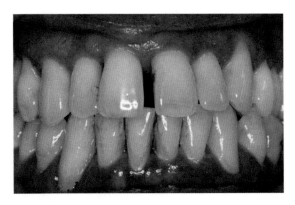

Figure 5.1 This patient presents with poor oral hygiene, plaque and calculus deposits, gingival bleeding, generalized gingival inflammation, and gingival recession. Clinical examination revealed generalized probing depths of 5–8 mm and alveolar bone loss affecting > 50% of the root length throughout the dentition. Her main concern is the appearance of the midline diastema, which has resulted from drifting of the upper incisors, notably tooth #8 (FDI 11). She wants something done about it! Cases such as this can be difficult to manage. It will probably not be possible to close the gap – orthodontics may not be appropriate even with a good outcome following the periodontal therapy. Expectation management is key – what is realistic to achieve must be explained from the outset

medical history that are particularly relevant to periodontal therapy are shown in Box 5.2. It is also useful to be aware of the patient's occupation, which can impact delivery of care (e.g., shift workers may find it difficult to attend appointments for treatment).

Box 5.2: Key aspects of medical history relevant to periodontal therapy

Smoking status

It is essential to record a full smoking history. This includes number of cigarettes per day and number of years of smoking. In the case of ex-smokers, record how many cigarettes they used to smoke per day, how many years they smoked for, and when they quit. All current smokers must be advised about the harmful aspects of smoking on periodontal health, and encouraged and supported in attempts to quit.

Diabetes

Diabetes, particularly if poorly controlled, increases the risk for periodontitis. Ask patients about their level of glycaemic control, and if they know their most recent glycated hemoglobin measurements (HbA1c).

Medical status

Conditions such as cardiovascular diseases, stroke, hematologic disorders, bleeding tendencies, cancer, liver disease, endocrine disorders, neurological problems, and infectious diseases may all influence the management strategy adopted for the patient. Liaison with the patient's medical physician may sometimes be necessary to obtain further information, to help the dentist plan the provision of dental care.

Medications

Certain medications are associated with drug-induced gingival overgrowth, such as some calcium channel blockers, phenytoin, and ciclosporin.

Bisphosphonate therapy (particularly intravenous therapy) increases the risk for osteonecrosis of the jaw.

Anticoagulants prolong bleeding, and will influence periodontal treatment decisions.

Corticosteroids (especially high doses) may influence immune responses and inflammation.

Allergy

This should include questions relating to medications, dental products (e.g., chlorhexidine, eugenol, and latex) as well as environmental allergens such as pollen.

Family history of periodontal disease

This is particularly relevant for younger individuals with suspected aggressive periodontitis, for which the key characteristics are advanced periodontitis (particularly in relation to age) in patients who are otherwise medically healthy, and who have a family history of periodontal disease.

PATIENT ASSESSMENT

PATIENT ASSESSMENT

Health History Form

ADA American Dental Association®
America's leading advocate for oral health

Email: _____ Today's Date: _____

As required by law, our office adheres to written policies and procedures to protect the privacy of information about you that we create, receive or maintain. Your answers are for our records only and will be kept confidential subject to applicable laws. Please note that you will be asked some questions about your responses to this questionnaire and there may be additional questions concerning your health. This information is vital to allow us to provide appropriate care for you. This office does not use this information to discriminate.

Name:			Home Phone: *Include area code*	Business/Cell Phone: *Include area code*
Last	*First*	*Middle*	( )	( )

Address:		City:	State:	Zip:
Mailing address				

Occupation:		Height:	Weight:	Date of Birth:	Sex: M F

SS# or Patient ID:	Emergency Contact:	Relationship:	Home Phone: *Include area code* ( )	Cell Phone: *Include area code* ( )

If you are completing this form for another person, what is your relationship to that person?

Your Name _____ *Relationship* _____

Do you have any of the following diseases or problems: (Check DK if you Don't Know the answer to the the question) Yes No DK

Active Tuberculosis.. ☐ ☐ ☐
Persistent cough greater than a 3 week duration............. ☐ ☐ ☐
Cough that produces blood.................................... ☐ ☐ ☐
Been exposed to anyone with tuberculosis.................... ☐ ☐ ☐

If you answer yes to any of the 4 items above, please stop and return this form to the receptionist.

Dental Information *For the following questions, please mark (X) your responses to the following questions.*

	Yes No DK		Yes No DK
Do your gums bleed when you brush or floss?	☐ ☐ ☐	Do you have earaches or neck pains?	☐ ☐ ☐
Are your teeth sensitive to cold, hot, sweets or pressure?	☐ ☐ ☐	Do you have any clicking, popping or discomfort in the jaw?	☐ ☐ ☐
Is your mouth dry?	☐ ☐ ☐	Do you brux or grind your teeth?	☐ ☐ ☐
Have you had any periodontal (gum) treatments?	☐ ☐ ☐	Do you have sores or ulcers in your mouth?	☐ ☐ ☐
Have you ever had orthodontic (braces) treatment?	☐ ☐ ☐	Do you wear dentures or partials?	☐ ☐ ☐
Have you had any problems associated with previous dental treatment?	☐ ☐ ☐	Do you participate in active recreational activities?	☐ ☐ ☐
Is your home water supply fluoridated?	☐ ☐ ☐	Have you ever had a serious injury to your head or mouth?	☐ ☐ ☐
Do you drink bottled or filtered water?	☐ ☐ ☐	Date of your last dental exam:	
If yes, how often? *Circle one:* DAILY / WEEKLY / OCCASIONALLY		What was done at that time?	
Are you currently experiencing dental pain or discomfort?	☐ ☐ ☐	Date of last dental x-rays:	

What is the reason for your dental visit today?

How do you feel about your smile?

Medical Information *Please mark (X) your response to indicate if you have or have not had any of the following diseases or problems.*

	Yes No DK		Yes No DK
Are you now under the care of a physician?	☐ ☐ ☐	Have you had a serious illness, operation or been hospitalized in the past 5 years?	☐ ☐ ☐
Physician Name:	Phone: *Include area code* ( )	If yes, what was the illness or problem?	
Address/City/State/Zip:		Are you taking or have you recently taken any prescription or over the counter medicine(s)?	☐ ☐ ☐
Are you in good health?	☐ ☐ ☐	If so, please list all, including vitamins, natural or herbal preparations and/or dietary supplements:	
Has there been any change in your general health within the past year?	☐ ☐ ☐	_____	
If yes, what condition is being treated?		_____	
Date of last physical exam:		_____	

© 2012 American Dental Association
Form S500

Figure 5.2 Health History Form from the American Dental Association – a great example of a comprehensive patient self-complete medical history form that is then reviewed and discussed by the clinician to ensure that full information about the patient's medical status is obtained. Copyright © 2013 American Dental Association. All rights reserved. (Reprinted with permission)

PATIENT ASSESSMENT

Medical Information *Please mark (X) your response to indicate if you have or have not had any of the following diseases or problems.*

	Yes	No	DK		Yes	No	DK
(Check DK if you Don't Know the answer to the question)				Do you use controlled substances (drugs)?	☐	☐	☐
Do you wear contact lenses?	☐	☐	☐	Do you use tobacco (smoking, snuff, chew, bidis)?	☐	☐	☐

Joint Replacement. Have you had an orthopedic total joint (hip, knee, elbow, finger) replacement? ☐ ☐ ☐

Date: _____ If yes, have you had any complications? _____

If so, how interested are you in stopping?
Circle one: VERY / SOMEWHAT / NOT INTERESTED

Do you drink alcoholic beverages? ☐ ☐ ☐

Are you taking or scheduled to begin taking an antiresorptive agent (like Fosamax®, Actonel®, Atelvia, Boniva®, Reclast, Prolia) for osteoporosis or Paget's disease? ☐ ☐ ☐

If yes, how much alcohol did you drink in the last 24 hours? _____

If yes, how much do you typically drink in a week? _____

Since 2001, were you treated or are you presently scheduled to begin treatment with an antiresorptive agent (like Aredia®, Zometa®, XGEVA) for bone pain, hypercalcemia or skeletal complications resulting from Paget's disease, multiple myeloma or metastatic cancer? ☐ ☐ ☐

Date Treatment began: _____

WOMEN ONLY Are you:
Pregnant? ☐ ☐ ☐
Number of weeks: _____
Taking birth control pills or hormonal replacement? ☐ ☐ ☐
Nursing? ☐ ☐ ☐

Allergies. Are you allergic to or have you had a reaction to:

To all yes responses, specify type of reaction.	Yes	No	DK		Yes	No	DK
Local anesthetics _____	☐	☐	☐	Metals _____	☐	☐	☐
Aspirin _____	☐	☐	☐	Latex (rubber) _____	☐	☐	☐
Penicillin or other antibiotics _____	☐	☐	☐	Iodine _____	☐	☐	☐
Barbiturates, sedatives, or sleeping pills _____	☐	☐	☐	Hay fever/seasonal _____	☐	☐	☐
Sulfa drugs _____	☐	☐	☐	Animals _____	☐	☐	☐
Codeine or other narcotics _____	☐	☐	☐	Food _____	☐	☐	☐
				Other _____	☐	☐	☐

Please mark (X) your response to indicate if you have or have not had any of the following diseases or problems.

	Yes	No	DK		Yes	No	DK		Yes	No	DK
Artificial (prosthetic) heart valve	☐	☐	☐	Autoimmune disease	☐	☐	☐	Glaucoma	☐	☐	☐
Previous infective endocarditis	☐	☐	☐	Rheumatoid arthritis	☐	☐	☐	Hepatitis, jaundice or liver disease	☐	☐	☐
Damaged valves in transplanted heart	☐	☐	☐	Systemic lupus erythematosus	☐	☐	☐	Epilepsy	☐	☐	☐
Congenital heart disease (CHD)				Asthma	☐	☐	☐	Fainting spells or seizures	☐	☐	☐
Unrepaired, cyanotic CHD	☐	☐	☐	Bronchitis	☐	☐	☐	Neurological disorders If yes, specify:	☐	☐	☐
Repaired (completely) in last 6 months	☐	☐	☐	Emphysema	☐	☐	☐	Sleep disorder	☐	☐	☐
Repaired CHD with residual defects	☐	☐	☐	Sinus trouble	☐	☐	☐	Do you snore?	☐	☐	☐
				Tuberculosis	☐	☐	☐	Mental health disorders Specify:	☐	☐	☐

Except for the conditions listed above, antibiotic prophylaxis is no longer recommended for any other form of CHD.

	Yes	No	DK		Yes	No	DK		Yes	No	DK
				Cancer/Chemotherapy/ Radiation Treatment	☐	☐	☐	Recurrent Infections Type of infection:	☐	☐	☐
Cardiovascular disease	☐	☐	☐	Chest pain upon exertion	☐	☐	☐				
Angina	☐	☐	☐	Mitral valve prolapse	☐	☐	☐	Kidney problems	☐	☐	☐
Arteriosclerosis	☐	☐	☐	Pacemaker	☐	☐	☐	Chronic pain	☐	☐	☐
								Night sweats	☐	☐	☐
Congestive heart failure	☐	☐	☐	Rheumatic fever	☐	☐	☐	Diabetes Type I or II	☐	☐	☐
Damaged heart valves	☐	☐	☐	Rheumatic heart disease	☐	☐	☐	Eating disorder	☐	☐	☐	Osteoporosis	☐	☐	☐
Heart attack	☐	☐	☐	Abnormal bleeding	☐	☐	☐	Malnutrition	☐	☐	☐	Persistent swollen glands in neck	☐	☐	☐
Heart murmur	☐	☐	☐	Anemia	☐	☐	☐	Gastrointestinal disease	☐	☐	☐				
Low blood pressure	☐	☐	☐	Blood transfusion If yes, date:	☐	☐	☐	G.E. Reflux/persistent heartburn	☐	☐	☐	Severe headaches/ migraines	☐	☐	☐
High blood pressure	☐	☐	☐	Hemophilia	☐	☐	☐	Ulcers	☐	☐	☐	Severe or rapid weight loss	☐	☐	☐
Other congenital heart defects	☐	☐	☐	AIDS or HIV infection	☐	☐	☐	Thyroid problems	☐	☐	☐	Sexually transmitted disease	☐	☐	☐
				Arthritis	☐	☐	☐	Stroke	☐	☐	☐	Excessive urination	☐	☐	☐

	Yes	No	DK
Has a physician or previous dentist recommended that you take antibiotics prior to your dental treatment?	☐	☐	☐

Name of physician or dentist making recommendation: _____ Phone: *Include area code* ( )

Do you have any disease, condition, or problem not listed above that you think I should know about? ☐ ☐ ☐
Please explain:

NOTE: Both doctor and patient are encouraged to discuss any and all relevant patient health issues prior to treatment.
I certify that I have read and understand the above and that the information given on this form is accurate. I understand the importance of a truthful health history and that my dentist and his/her staff will rely on this information for treating me. I acknowledge that my questions, if any, about inquiries set forth above have been answered to my satisfaction. I will not hold my dentist, or any other member of his/her staff, responsible for any action they take or do not take because of errors or omissions that I may have made in the completion of this form.

Signature of Patient/Legal Guardian: _____ Date: _____

Signature of Dentist: _____ Date: _____

FOR COMPLETION BY DENTIST
Comments: _____

Figure 5.2 *(continued)*

The dental history should also be recorded. In relation to periodontal treatment, it is important to ascertain whether the patient has previously received periodontal therapy, and what form it took. Was surgical or nonsurgical treatment provided? How many episodes of instrumentation were performed? Was anesthesia used? How many appointments has the patient attended for periodontal therapy, including maintenance care? Or, is the patient presenting for the first time for periodontal therapy? It is also important to be aware of other planned dental treatment, such as restorative care, provision of fixed or removable prostheses, endodontics, orthodontics or implant therapy.

Clinical examination

It is necessary to perform a complete oral and dental examination. Extraoral assessment should focus on the lymph nodes, temporomandibular joints, and muscles of mastication. Intraoral examination must include a full dental charting (teeth present, caries, restorations, and tooth surface loss) as well as examination of the oral soft tissues (lips, tongue, palate, buccal mucosa, floor of mouth, and oropharynx).

Make an assessment of the level of oral hygiene, particularly focusing on plaque deposits at the gingival margin and interproximally, as well as the presence of calculus. Note sites at which oral hygiene is suboptimal, and consider if this is due to patient ineffectiveness (e.g., the patient may not be performing daily hygiene in these regions, or may be using the wrong oral hygiene device), or is due to local factors that make daily hygiene difficult in these regions (e.g., as a result of the presence of overhanging margins of restorations). Evaluate the gingival tissues for evidence of inflammation (characterized by redness and swelling), or other pathologies (e.g., drug induced gingival overgrowth). Drying of the tissues is important to improve visibility when examining the gingival tissues.

The cornerstone of the periodontal examination is periodontal probing, and involves the use of a periodontal probe. Periodontal probing is essential for periodontal diagnosis, treatment planning, and monitoring, and is the only reliable method available for detecting periodontal pockets. Periodontal pockets cannot be visualized on radiographs. A schematic representation of a periodontal pocket is shown in Figure 5.3.

Although periodontal probing is often regarded as a simple procedure to perform, it is actually technically challenging and prone to error. The recorded probing depths can be affected by multiple factors including:

- probe position, angulation, and orientation
- force (pressure) applied
- probe diameter
- probe tip sharpness/bluntness
- clarity of probe markings and visibility of the site
- presence of blood, saliva, plaque, all of which can obscure probe markings
- presence of calculus (supra- or subgingival)
- margins of restorations

The force that should be applied when probing is generally considered to be around 0.25 Newtons (Hefti, 1997). This can be difficult to assess, but is typically the amount of force required to depress the skin on the pad of the thumb by about 1 mm with a periodontal probe.

Probing depths should be recorded at 6 sites per tooth (Figure 5.4). A systematic approach is essential to ensure that no sites are missed, and that the recording of the probing depths either onto paper records or into a computer system is accurate. A common method is to record probing depths as follows:

1. Buccal surfaces of upper arch (from right to left)

2. Palatal surfaces of upper arch (from left to right)

3. Buccal surfaces of lower arch (from right to left)

4. Lingual surfaces of lower arch (from left to right).

The probe should be inserted into the pocket, approximately parallel to the long axis of the tooth and "walked" around the tooth to record the probing depths. At interproximal sites, the probe will need to be angled slightly to ensure that the probe tip is at the depth of the pocket, which is typically below the contact point.

Record the probing depth measurements either onto a paper form, or into a computerized recording system. The most important aspect of the chart is that it should permit site-by-site comparisons of probing depths recorded at sequential probing examinations over time (e.g., so pre- and posttreatment measurements can be

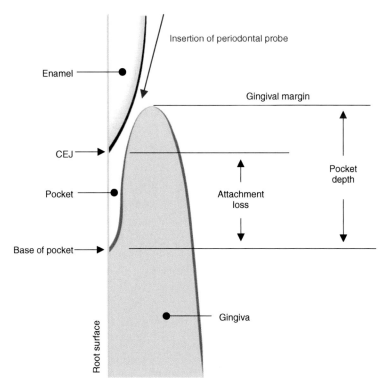

Figure 5.3 Schematic representation of a periodontal pocket. The probe is inserted to the depth of the pocket, and the measured probing depth is the distance from the free gingival margin to the probe tip, which is assumed to be at the base of the pocket. In inflamed tissues, the probe tends to penetrate the tissues at the base of the pocket, resulting in bleeding on probing, and also a higher measured probing depth (compared to the true pocket depth). Following treatment, resolution of inflammation results in shrinkage of the gingival tissues and greater resistance of the tissues at the base of the pocket to penetration by the probe. Both of these factors result in reduced probing depths following treatment. Whereas the reference point for measuring probing depth is the gingival margin, the reference point for measuring attachment loss is the CEJ. It may often be difficult to locate the CEJ, particularly in patients presenting with gingival inflammation, and for this reason, probing depths are the more useful measure for assessing periodontal status and response to treatment. CEJ: cemento-enamel junction. (*Source*: Preshaw et al., 2012. Reproduced with permission of Springer)

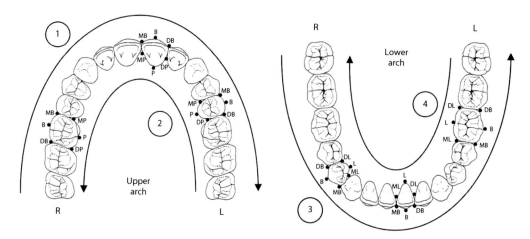

Figure 5.4 Follow a systematic approach when performing periodontal probing. 1: probe all the buccal sites in the upper arch, from right to left, starting at the disto-buccal aspect of the last standing molar. It is convenient to pause at the midline and call out bleeding on probing scores for the buccal aspects of the first quadrant (upper right quadrant) before progressing to probing the buccal aspects of the upper left quadrant. Call out the bleeding on probing scores for the upper left after completing the upper left probing. 2: after completing the buccal measurements, record the palatal probing depths in the maxilla, this time from left to right (again, it is useful to pause in the midline to call out bleeding scores before proceeding to completing the probing assessments at the right side). Repeat the process in the mandible: buccal first from right to left, and then lingual from left to right. Probe placement locations at six sites are shown on selected teeth. MB: mesio-buccal; B: buccal (i.e., mid-buccal); DB: disto-buccal; MP: mesio-palatal; P: palatal (i.e., mid-palatal); DP: disto-palatal; ML: mesio-lingual; L: lingual (i.e., mid-lingual); DL: disto-lingual

viewed on a site-by-site basis). An example of a paper-based probing chart is shown in Figure 5.5 and more thoughts about periodontal probing are presented in Box 5.3.

During the probing procedure, also measure recession, if present, at each site, as the distance from the CEJ to the gingival margin. BOP should be recorded as present/absent at each site following probing. In patients with minimally inflamed tissues, there may be very little bleeding, in which case it may be reasonable to wait until the midline has been reached in the probing sequence, and then look back over the probed quadrant to identify any isolated bleeding sites. On the other hand, in patients with extensive gingival inflammation (Figure 5.6), there may be profuse bleeding immediately after each site is probed, and in this case, it is more accurate to record BOP scores immediately after probing each site.

The presence of furcations should be assessed, using a curved furcation probe. Every furcation entrance should be checked: for maxillary

molars, there are three potential furcations to assess (mid-buccal, mesio-palatal, disto-palatal) whereas for mandibular molars, there are two potential furcations to assess (mid-buccal, mid-lingual).

It may also be necessary to assess the occlusion in certain cases, and study models may be indicated. Clinical photographs can also be a useful component of the initial patient assessment.

IDENTIFYING SITES TO TREAT

Decisions about which teeth to retain and which to extract, or which sites to perform root surface debridement (RSD) at, can be very difficult to make. The main reason for the difficulty is that we cannot see into the future; we do not know which sites will progress, which sites will respond well to treatment, or whether the patient will be able to maintain compromised teeth.

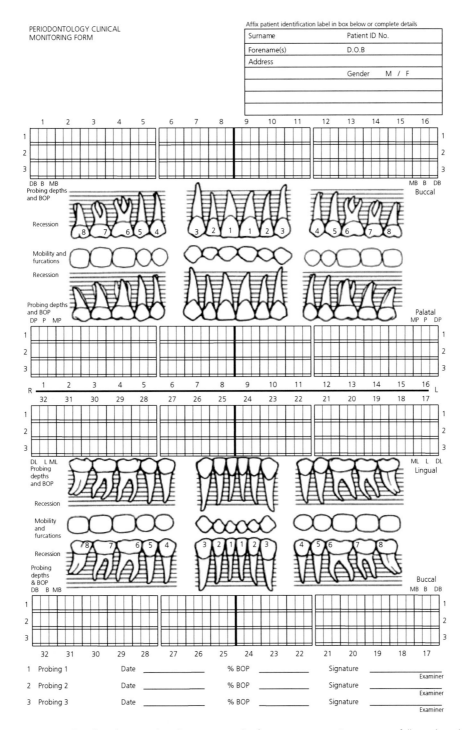

Figure 5.5 Paper recording form for periodontal assessment. This form permits up to 3 consecutive full mouth probing records to be made, allowing for site-by-site comparison in changes in probing depths that occur following treatment. Bleeding on probing can be recorded by circling the probing depth measurements (or, on this form, by shading in the small rectangle under each probing depth measurement). Recession can be drawn onto the form, as well as indications of mobility and furcation involvement

Box 5.3: Periodontal probing – so much to think about!

The 6 sites versus Walk that Probe!

Recording probing depths at six sites per tooth (MB, B, DB, ML, L, DL) as shown in Figure 5.4 is standard throughout the world. These sites have been chosen because most of the time, they coincide with the locations of the deepest pockets around a tooth. The MB, DB, ML and DL locations are aiming to identify pockets underneath the contact points, which tend to be the areas at which the deepest pockets are located. And, the B and L (i.e., mid-buccal and mid-lingual) measurements at molars tend to coincide with areas of furcation involvement.

The question often arises: should I only insert the probe at exactly those 6 locations when I examine a patient, or should I "walk" the probe around the entire circumference of the tooth?

The answer is that we walk that probe! We walk the probe around the entire circumference of the tooth so that we can find the deepest probing depth measurements around the tooth, because that is what we are most interested in. We then use our clinical skill and judgment to record the deepest measurement at a particular region of the tooth into the most relevant (i.e., closest) of the six standard locations.

What else do we assess with a periodontal probe?

The periodontal probe is a pretty useful tool. We measure probing depths with it and elicit bleeding on probing as an indicator of inflammation. We wipe it along the tooth surface as we proceed with our examination to identify plaque (keep some gauze handy to wipe it clean so you can still read the markings on the probe). We use it to detect the presence of calculus and make assessments of root morphology. All of these factors are used to help us determine which sites to treat and how to treat them.

A research study reports a mean probing depth reduction of 1.2 mm… that doesn't sound like much!

When we see an individual patient, and provide periodontal treatment, we naturally focus on the deep sites and the response to treatment at those individual sites. We may see a particular pocket reduce from 6 mm to 4 mm, or from 8 mm to 5 mm. Yet, when we read the research literature, much smaller probing depth reductions seem to be reported – why is this?

The answer is that most research studies report mean (i.e., average) probing depth reductions following treatment, across all sites. If a full mouth mean change is reported, this includes every site in the mouth, including the sites that were deep prior to treatment, as well as those that were shallow prior to treatment. Most patients with periodontitis have a mix of deep sites and shallow sites, including sites that may be 3 mm or less prior to treatment. We don't expect those shallow sites to particularly change following therapy. Therefore, when calculating a mean probing depth reduction across the entire dentition, those shallow sites which don't change much have the effect of "diluting" or "reducing"' the magnitude of the probing depth reductions that occurred at the sites that were deep prior to treatment. Many studies nowadays stratify the analysis according to initial probing depth, for example, they might only report the probing depth reductions at sites that were 5 mm or greater prior to treatment, and ignore any changes at the sites that were 4 mm or less prior to treatment.

As an example, consider the patient shown in Figure 5.7. This patient attended for the first time in 2004 (Figure 5.7a), and a diagnosis of chronic periodontitis was reached. The treatment strategy involved personalized oral hygiene instruction, and ultrasonic RSD. No decisions were made about extractions, other than noting the poor prognosis of several of the teeth, including the first molars, notably #19 (FDI 36). This tooth responded positively to vitality testing, and the decision was made to retain the tooth. Further radiographs were obtained in 2007 (Figure 5.7b) and 2010 (Figure 5.7c) and throughout this period, the patient continued to receive periodontal maintenance care. The patient was able to achieve a high standard of oral hygiene, with excellent plaque control and minimal gingival inflammation, as can be seen in the clinical image

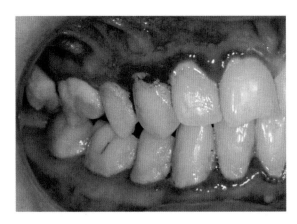

Figure 5.6 A new patient presenting for periodontal treatment for the first time. Initial inspection reveals extremely poor oral hygiene, abundant plaque and calculus deposits, extensive gingival inflammation and spontaneous gingival bleeding. Accurate periodontal probing will be difficult to perform because of the abundant plaque and calculus and the high probability of profuse bleeding after probing at each site. Nonetheless, an effort should be made to complete a full probing chart prior to commencing any treatment – it will take time (longer than usual!), with the need to remove plaque from the probe with a gauze swab after each probing measurement, and washing/aspiration and drying of the tissues to improve visibility

obtained in 2010 (Figure 5.7d). Over this six-year period, the periodontal condition remained stable, there was no particular evidence of disease progression, and tooth #19 (FDI 36) remained vital, functional, and symptom-free.

How many clinicians would have recommended extraction of tooth #19 (FDI 36) when the patient first presented in 2004? What other treatment options might have been considered? For example, extraction and replacement with an implant could have been considered, or alternatively, periodontal surgery involving hemisection of the tooth and removal of the distal root (and probably also endodontic treatment) could have been performed. Yet, in this case, the simplest treatment option (i.e., nonsurgical management involving RSD, oral hygiene instruction and long-term periodontal maintenance care) proved to be highly effective. Clearly, the patient was very compliant, but if the patient had not been able to maintain such a high level of plaque control, then the surgical options (e.g., implant placement or hemisection) would not have been indicated anyway. Review of the clinical chart for this patient reveals that the probing depth at the distal aspect of #19 (FDI 36) was 10 mm in 2004, 8 mm in 2007 and 5 mm in 2010.

This case highlights the difficulties that clinicians can face when deciding how to treat a patient with periodontitis. The "biological model" of periodontal treatment that was advocated by Kieser (see Chapter 1) suggests that the treatment response is assessed by evaluating the soft tissue changes that occur following therapy. Therefore, our treatment outcomes should be based on soft tissue parameters (e.g., probing depths, BOP). Kieser advocated a pragmatic, staged treatment strategy in which RSD is performed with ultrasonic instruments, adopting a light-touch approach to minimize removal of tooth substance, while at the same time disrupting and removing biofilm (as well as removing plaque-retentive features such as calculus). It is important that the patient knows that one episode of RSD is not the end of their periodontal treatment – most patients will undergo various episodes of RSD interspersed with longer periods of periodontal maintenance care, with a strong emphasis on optimized self-performed plaque control at all times.

Probing depths

The biological model of periodontal therapy indicates that periodontal treatment should not follow a "cook book" approach. In other words, just because a pocket is x mm deep, this should not result in a treatment decision that is taken in isolation from all the other factors that are relevant for that tooth (such as BOP, furcations, mobility, occlusion, vitality, endodontic status, presence of restorations, presence of dentures, and distribution of teeth in the dentition). Probing depths are, of course, extremely important when deciding which sites to treat, but clearly, multiple factors should be taken into consideration when planning periodontal therapy, and a "one size fits all" approach is unlikely to be

PATIENT ASSESSMENT

PATIENT ASSESSMENT

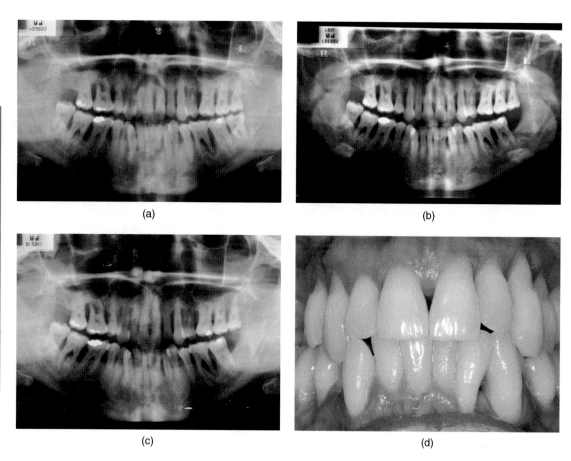

(a)

(b)

(c)

(d)

Figure 5.7 Radiographs obtained in 2004 (a), 2007 (b) and 2010 (c) which reveal that, although the patient presented with advanced periodontitis and generalized advanced alveolar bone loss with multiple vertical defects, over the course of 6 years of non-surgical periodontal therapy (episodes of RSD and OHI interspersed with periods of periodontal maintenance care) bone levels remained reasonably stable with no particular evidence of disease progression, even at compromised teeth such as #19 (FDI 36). The patient's compliance with the periodontal therapy and excellent plaque control are evident in the clinical image (d) obtained in 2010

successful in all cases. The therapy should be individualized to the clinical situation and the needs and wishes of the patient, taking all the relevant factors into account.

It has been shown in many classic studies of periodontal therapy that nonsurgical periodontal instrumentation is a highly effective procedure that results in improvements in plaque and bleeding scores, and reductions in probing depths (Badersten et al., 1981; Badersten et al., 1984; Badersten et al., 1985; Claffey et al., 1990; Lindhe et al., 1989; Pihlstrom et al., 1983). These early studies found that there is no initial depth of

pocket above which nonsurgical management is not effective – in other words, even at sites with very deep pockets, there can be a benefit of nonsurgical instrumentation.

Over the years, a large number of studies have assessed the clinical response to nonsurgical therapy, and these have been extensively reviewed (Cobb, 2002). Reductions in probing depths following therapy result from resolution of inflammation (i.e., a soft tissue response), characterized by shrinkage of the periodontal tissues and increased tissue resistance to penetration by the probe at the base of the pocket. The

Table 5.1 Typical expected outcomes following periodontal non-surgical therapy, according to initial probing depth

Initial probing depth	Expected changes in probing depth and attachment level
1–3 mm	Mean probing depth reduction: 0.03 mm Mean loss in attachment level: −0.34 mm
4–6 mm	Mean probing depth reduction: 1.29 mm Mean gain in attachment level: 0.55 mm
7 mm and greater	Mean probing depth reduction: 2.16 mm Mean gain in attachment level: 1.19 mm

Data from Cobb (1996) and Cobb (2002).

typical probing depth reductions and changes in attachment level that have been reported in clinical studies are presented, stratified according to baseline probing depth, in Table 5.1 (Cobb, 1996; Cobb 2002). Of course, these are mean changes in probing depths, whereas in normal clinical practice, we do not calculate mean probing depths across the entire dentition. Instead, we assess the outcomes of therapy on a site-by-site basis, by measuring probing depths pre- and posttreatment. In other words, clinically relevant changes in probing depths are used to assess treatment outcomes on a site-by-site basis as opposed to changes in mean probing depths across the entire dentition. What constitutes a clinically relevant change is a matter for debate, but most operators appear to agree that a probing depth reduction at a particular site of at least 2 mm is a clinically relevant finding, whereas a change of 1 mm could more simply be a result of measurement error (Hefti, 1997; Osborn et al., 1992). Box 5.3 expands further on interpreting probing depth reductions that are reported in research studies in comparison to probing depth reductions that we see in our individual patients following treatment.

The decision about whether to perform instrumentation at a particular site is also influenced by the phase of treatment that the patient is in. For example, in the patient shown in Figure 5.7, the probing depth at the distal aspect of #19 (FDI 36) was 5 mm in 2010. Most clinicians would agree that a 5 mm pocket requires instrumentation, but in this case, the probing depth had already reduced from 10 mm in 2004, representing an excellent response to treatment. By 2010, the patient was enrolled in an ongoing periodontal maintenance program that included visits with the dental hygienist every 3 months for ultrasonic instrumentation subgingivally throughout the dentition, including the pocket at the distal of #19 (FDI 36). The aim when treating this site was the disruption of the subgingival biofilm as a means by which to control inflammation in the periodontal tissues. Since then, the pocket has continued to be stable, with a 5 mm probing depth, and this can be considered a highly satisfactory outcome that warrants no further intervention other than the ongoing periodontal maintenance care. It would not be in the patient's best interests in this case to try to "eliminate" the pocket by performing periodontal surgery to try to reduce the probing depth to, for example, 3 mm or less, because there is no indication to perform such a procedure (i.e., there are no active signs or symptoms that would justify such an approach), and performing surgery would not guarantee an improved outcome and could actually carry the risk of harm and potentially compromise the tooth.

Decisions about instrumentation are therefore complex – not only must we consider the probing depth, but also the phase of treatment, as well as other factors that affect the clinical situation. The reason for performing RSD is to reduce the bacterial challenge by disrupting and removing biofilm so that there is a resultant reduction in inflammation. As inflammation subsides, the tissues shrink, the pockets becomes shallower, and therefore easier to maintain, and are more accessible to clean. The pocket environment also alters as the pocket depth reduces so that the growth of less pathogenic species is favored – see Chapter 1.

Most clinicians would agree that RSD is required for sites of 5 mm or greater. Furthermore, RSD is required for all sites (regardless of depth) at which persistent inflammation is noted. For patients newly presenting with periodontal disease, full mouth ultrasonic RSD will typically be indicated, and, therefore, sites of less than 5 mm will be instrumented (e.g., sites of 2–4 mm). Although it has previously been reported in some studies that there is a "critical value" of probing depth, below which instrumentation could result in loss of attachment as a result of tissue damage and resultant inflammation (Lindhe et al., 1982), it is important to remember that these studies primarily utilized root planing rather than modern techniques of light-touch ultrasonic instrumentation. We advocate, therefore, that *all* probing depths may be treated with ultrasonic RSD, utilizing a gentle, light-touch approach, with correct selection of ultrasonic tips to ensure the best adaptation of the instrument according to the anatomical situation.

As a result of the initial periodontal therapy for a newly diagnosed patient, we hope that, with good oral hygiene, compliance, and effective RSD, there will be a generalized reduction in probing depths as a result of resolution of inflammation. This is a positive outcome, as shallower pockets are easier to maintain. It is important not to perform posttreatment probing too soon after the initial therapy, and we recommend that posttreatment probing is performed at 3 months. There is evidence that, although the majority of resolution of inflammation is complete by 3 months, there can be further improvements as the tissues mature and stabilize for up to 9 months following the initial therapy (Badersten et al., 1984). Reevaluation of probing depths is an extremely important part of periodontal therapy, as the effectiveness of the therapy and the nature of the subsequent treatment are then decided. By probing earlier than 3 months following initial therapy, there will have been insufficient time for resolution of inflammation to fully occur, and, therefore, decisions about future treatment need may be incorrectly made because probing depths are still in the process of reducing as inflammation resolves.

Bleeding on probing (BOP)

BOP is routinely assessed to measure the degree of gingival and periodontal inflammation. BOP can arise from the probe penetrating the tissues at the base of the pocket, or from traumatizing the epithelial lining of the pocket (which may well be ulcerated) at any point from the gingival margin to the depth of the pocket. It is, therefore, very difficult (and probably not relevant) to try and discriminate between bleeding from the base of the pocket or from the gingival tissues. Furthermore, the presence of BOP at isolated sites is not a particularly good indicator of risk for future disease progression (Lang et al., 1986), whereas absence of BOP is a good indicator of periodontal health and tissue stability (Chapple, 1997; Lang et al., 1990). However, BOP is definitely a useful parameter to record, as it provides an indication of the degree of inflammation in the gingival and periodontal tissues. It is also a clinical parameter that is very relevant to patients, who often may complain of bleeding gums (e.g., when brushing their teeth, or on waking in the morning). In smokers, gingival bleeding may be reduced because of the effect of smoking on the gingival vasculature, and on quitting, many smokers report a transient increase in gingival bleeding.

Although BOP at isolated sites is not a strong indicator of increased risk for future attachment loss, persistent BOP plus an increase in probing depth is an indicator of increased risk. For example, in patients who received periodontal maintenance care for 42 months after initial periodontal therapy, plaque scores demonstrated low predictability for future disease progression and bleeding scores showed modest predictive values, whereas increases in probing depths in the maintenance phase, particularly if associated with BOP, showed the highest predictive value for future occurrence of attachment loss

(Claffey et al., 1990). It has also been identified that persistent BOP during the periodontal maintenance phase (i.e., as identified at successive maintenance visits) is a strong indicator of risk for ongoing progression of periodontitis (Schatzle et al., 2003).

BOP should be recorded, therefore, whenever a full periodontal probing chart is completed, and a high level of suspicion should be placed on sites that, in the maintenance phase of care, show evidence of increasing probing depth and BOP, as these are the sites at greatest risk for future attachment loss.

FACTORS TO ASSESS AT DISEASE SITES

As outlined above, the probing depth and presence or absence of BOP are generally the two most important factors to consider when deciding to perform treatment, and deciding what kind of therapy should be undertaken. Many other factors also influence treatment decisions, however, and consideration of these factors is also important in helping to select the correct instrument to use at a particular site. Some of these factors are considered in the following text, but it is important to remember that this list can never be exhaustive, and the clinician will need to make their own decisions based on the clinical situation that they are faced with.

Pocket anatomy

The anatomy of the pocket will influence decisions about which instrument to use. It is impossible to make a detailed assessment of pocket anatomy (the pocket being a soft tissue structure) but we can assess the depth of the pocket with the periodontal probe (i.e., record probing depths) and also the tightness of the gingival tissues surrounding the teeth. Pretreatment, when the tissues are inflamed, it is generally quite easy to insert instruments into the pocket. During the maintenance phase, when there has been resolution of inflammation following the initial therapy, the gingival tissues may form a tighter cuff around the tooth, making it more difficult to insert instruments. It is important, therefore, to select the correct instrument type to avoid traumatizing the soft tissues. Manufacturers of ultrasonic instruments produce a variety of tips with different lengths, diameter and curvature. Slim and ultraslim tips offer the advantage of providing good tactile feedback about the root surface anatomy and presence of tooth deposits within the subgingival environment. The curvature of the root surface should also be taken into consideration when selecting the most appropriate tip to debride a particular site, to achieve maximal contact between the active area of the tip and the root surface (see Chapter 4).

Types of deposits

During initial periodontal therapy, there are likely to be heavy calculus deposits that are tenaciously adherent to the tooth surface (both supra- and subgingival), and the gingival tissues are likely to be noticeably inflamed. On the other hand, during the maintenance phase of therapy (i.e., once the initial therapy has been completed, and the patient is returning for supportive care), the tissues will be less inflamed and more tightly adapted to the tooth surface. At this phase of therapy, the tooth deposits that will require removal will primarily be supra- and subgingival plaque deposits, and a minimal amount of calculus (Badersten et al., 1981; Flemmig et al., 1998). These factors are highly relevant to the choice of tip that should be utilized, as different instrument efficacies are needed for debridement during the initial therapy and during supportive periodontal therapy. In general terms, the tip should be selected to achieve the most efficient debridement of the root surface, with consideration given to the anatomy of the root surface, the type of deposit and the power level. For heavy calculus deposits that are typically

PATIENT ASSESSMENT

Table 5.2 Furcation classification scoring systems

4 point furcation scoring system proposed by Glickman (1953) *(and the scoring system used in this book)*

Grade 1 furcation	Incipient furcation involvement in which there is pocket formation into the "flute" of the furcation, but no horizontal loss of attachment into the furcation itself
Grade 2 furcation	Loss of attachment into the furcation, but not completely through to the opposite side of the tooth, that is, is a cul-de-sac furcation involvement
Grade 3 furcation	Horizontal "through-and-through" involvement in which the lesion extends across the entire width of the furcation
Grade 4 furcation	Same as a Grade 3 furcation, but with gingival recession that has rendered the furcation region clearly visible on clinical examination

3-point furcation scoring system proposed by Hamp et al. (1975) *(not used in this book)*

Grade 1 furcation	Horizontal loss of attachment into the furcation of < 3 mm (~1/3 the tooth width)
Grade 2 furcation	Horizontal loss of attachment into the furcation of > 3 mm (or approximately 1/3 the tooth width), but does not pass completely through the furcation, that is, is a cul-de-sac furcation involvement
Grade 3 furcation	Horizontal "through-and-through" involvement in which the lesion extends across the entire width of the furcation

encountered at initial therapy, standard-diameter tips are generally indicated for efficient reduction and removal of the calculus, and they can be introduced into pockets with relative ease when the tissues are inflamed. Slim and ultraslim tips are generally indicated for removal and disruption of the plaque biofilm and smaller calculus deposits, and are likely to be particularly useful in the maintenance phase of periodontal therapy when the tissues are more tightly adapted around the tooth (see Chapter 4).

Furcations, concavities, grooves, and ridges

Teeth have complicated root morphologies, particularly when periodontal attachment loss exposes the furcation region of multirooted teeth (Cattabriga et al., 2000). The presence of furcations should be assessed, classified and recorded as part of the periodontal examination. The two most commonly used furcation classification systems are presented in Table 5.2 (Glickman, 1953; Hamp et al., 1975). In this book, we will use the four-point furcation classification system that was originally proposed by Glickman in 1953.

With reference to the anatomy of furcation entrances, it has been reported that 81% of furcation entrances in maxillary and mandibular first molars are ≤ 1 mm wide, and 58% are ≤ 0.75 mm wide, whereas the width of the blades of hand instruments was typically in the range 0.75–1.10 mm (Bower, 1979a). Similar findings were also reported in Chinese maxillary molars, in which the majority of furcation entrances in second molars were smaller than the width of a manual curette (Hou et al., 1994). More recently, it was reported that 19% of furcation entrances in extracted molar teeth (maxillary and mandibular) were < 0.60 mm whereas 75% of hand instrument blades were wider than this (dos Santos et al., 2009).

In mandibular molars, the furcation entrance is usually narrower than the central region of the furcation (Figure 5.8). For example, in mandibular first molars, the furcal aspects of the mesial and distal roots are generally concave (with mean concavity depths of 0.7 mm at the mesial root and 0.5 mm at the distal root), resulting in the central region of the furcation being, on average, 1.2 mm wider than the furcation entrance

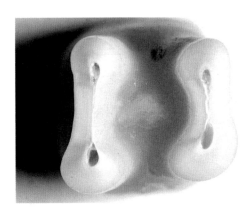

Figure 5.8 Mandibular first molar (#19, FDI 36) which has been sectioned at the mid-root level to reveal that the central part of the furcation is much wider than either of the furcation entrances

(Bower, 1979b). The same research identified that the furcal aspect of maxillary first molar roots is concave in 94% of mesio-buccal roots, 31% of disto-buccal roots and 17% of palatal roots.

The complicated anatomy of the furcation makes these locations very difficult to debride. The narrow entrance to the furcation is a particular concern. Narrow-diameter, curved ultrasonic tips will provide the greatest opportunity for instrumenting these regions. *In vitro* studies of extracted teeth have confirmed that ultrasonic instruments are effective in removing calculus from within furcations (Takacs et al., 1993), and are more effective and time efficient in debriding the furcation region than hand instruments (Oda and Ishikawa, 1989; Scott et al., 1999). Ultrasonic furcation tips were also shown to be more effective in calculus removal than conventional ultrasonic tips or hand instruments particularly in deeper furcations at which the horizontal probing depth was > 2 mm (Sugaya et al., 2002).

Treatment studies have confirmed that clinically significant improvements can be realized following nonsurgical ultrasonic debridement of furcations (Del Peloso Ribeiro et al., 2007). In a comparison study of a single session of either hand scaling or ultrasonic instrumentation in six patients with 33 furcation-involved molars, in

Class II and III furcations, ultrasonic debridement was significantly more effective than hand scaling in decreasing counts of motile rods and spirochetes, and decreasing gingival crevicular fluid flow (there was no difference between the treatment modalities at Class I furcations) (Leon and Vogel, 1987). In a study of periodontally diseased mandibular molars that were scheduled for extraction, but which underwent periodontal instrumentation prior to being extracted, more calculus was removed by ultrasonic instruments than by hand instruments (more calculus was removed following open surgical procedures than closed, nonsurgical procedures) (Matia et al., 1986). These studies clearly support that ultrasonic instruments are effective in treating furcation-involved teeth, and provide better access and more efficient therapy than hand instruments.

Teeth often have concavities in the root surfaces; for example, it was reported that mesial concavities were present in 100% of maxillary first premolars evaluated (Booker and Loughlin, 1985). Grooves are also present at many locations, for example, around 80% of maxillary first premolars have a groove (buccal furcation groove) on the furcation surface of the buccal root (Gher and Vernino, 1980), and palatoradicular grooves are not an uncommon finding, particularly at the palatal aspect of maxillary lateral incisors. Ridges in cementum are also present at many teeth. Intermediate bifurcation ridges have been reported to be present in as many as 75% of mandibular molars; these are ridges of cementum that originate at the mesial surface of the distal root, cross the bifurcation, and continue to the mesial root (Burch and Hulen, 1974).

The anatomical complexities of root surfaces can therefore present considerable challenges for therapy. In broad terms, narrow-diameter, curved ultrasonic tips can be used to negotiate narrow grooves and furcation entrances more effectively than standard-diameter tips or manual instruments, and they provide better tactile feedback for the clinician about the root surface that is being instrumented than standard-diameter tips.

Presence of restorations

Crown margins are frequently located slightly subgingivally to optimize aesthetics. Other restorative materials including composite resins, glass ionomers and amalgams also frequently are located close to, or below the gingival margin, and in all these instances it is important to avoid damaging the margins of the restorations during periodontal therapy. In an *in vitro* study of the impact of ultrasonic instrumentation on buccal and lingual class V composite and amalgam restorations, it was found that there was no detrimental impact of either ultrasonic instrumentation or air polishing on marginal integrity or microleakage of the restorations (Gorfil et al., 1989). In a study of the effect of various piezoelectric ultrasonic scaler tips applied to restorative materials such as amalgam, composite and porcelain, it was reported that broader-diameter tips resulted in more surface roughness and chips in the restorative materials, as assessed by profilometry and stereomicroscopy (Arabaci et al., 2007). The impact of ultrasonic and sonic instruments on the surface roughness of tooth colored restorative materials including composite resins, glass ionomers and a compomer placed in class V cavities has also been reported (Lai et al., 2007). Surface roughness was assessed with a profilometer before and after instrumentation; instrumentation was performed with the instrument tip applied at 15° to the restoration surface for 60 seconds with water irrigation. Both the ultrasonic and sonic instruments resulted in significant increases in surface roughness of the majority of the tested materials. The glass ionomers demonstrated the greatest increases in surface roughness as a result of the instrumentation whereas the composite resins demonstrated the smallest increases. Further investigations of the impact of ultrasonics on the surface characteristics of composite resins revealed that both parallel and perpendicular orientations of the ultrasonic tip produced indentations in the composite surface, with a scattering of composite debris (Walmsley et al., 1997).

A comparison of the effect of manual (curettes), ultrasonic and sonic instruments on the surface characteristics of composite resins has been reported (Bjornson et al 1990). Composite resin specimens were instrumented for 45 strokes with the manual instrument, or for 60 seconds with either the ultrasonic or sonic instruments. It was reported that the manual instrument was applied at a force of 1 kg, after prior studies of the forces applied by five clinicians revealed a range of 0.2–1.0 kg being applied when root planing with manual instruments. The ultrasonic and sonic instruments were applied at a force of 25 g. Samples were assessed for weight reduction following treatment (indicating loss of material from the surface), particle/debris size, and scanning electron microscopy evaluation of the surface. It was found that the manual curette applied at a force typically encountered when root planing removed a significant amount of material and altered the surface profile of the composite samples. The ultrasonic and sonic scalers removed far less material, and the ultrasonic instrument in particular did not significantly alter the surface.

It is clear, therefore, that all periodontal instruments have the capacity to modify the surfaces of restorative materials (i.e., cause surface roughness), although there is evidence that ultrasonic instruments tend to be less damaging than manual (hand) instruments. Factors such as the hardness of the restorative material and the degree of force applied during instrumentation are relevant, and whichever instruments are used, care should be taken to avoid causing surface damage. On balance, it appears that ultrasonic instruments are the least likely to cause surface roughness in restorative materials, and the general principles of ultrasonic instrumentation (e.g., multiple light strokes, keeping the tip moving, not applying the tip directly against the restoration surface) should be utilized to minimize the likelihood of causing damage to restorative materials.

Location of gingival margin

The location of the gingival margin in relation to tooth deposits and/or restorations should also be evaluated when planning therapy. (Or, to put it another way, the location of tooth deposits in relation to the gingival margin should be considered.) Some ultrasonic tips are designed to be used purely in a supragingival location, and these are used for removal of heavy deposits of supragingival calculus, particularly in scaling procedures that have the aim of reducing the bulk of calculus present. Apart from these tips, most brands and designs of ultrasonic tips can be utilized at both supragingival and subgingival locations. In general terms, narrow-diameter ultrasonic tips are the preferred choice for subgingival debridement because they provide good tactile feedback regarding the surface being instrumented, they can access furcations and grooves better than standard-diameter tips, and they are less likely to cause soft or hard tissue trauma.

MEDICAL CONSIDERATIONS AND OTHER PATIENT FACTORS

As described earlier in this chapter, a full medical history should be recorded for all patients, and reviewed and updated at every visit. A number of medical considerations must be taken into account when considering periodontal therapy, and some issues that are relevant to all forms of periodontal treatment are described in Box 5.2. Other specific scenarios that may be encountered in some patients will be considered now.

Pacemakers

A degree of controversy exists within the dental literature in relation to the use of magnetostrictive ultrasonic scalers in patients with implanted pacemakers. The theoretical risk relates to electromagnetic interference (EMI), which describes the effect of an electromagnetic field on the operation of an implanted heart rhythm device (pacemaker). EMI occurs when signals from an electromagnetic field (e.g., as created by electrical and magnetic devices) temporarily interfere with the pacemaker, which may interpret the electromagnetic signals as coming from the heart and respond by withholding its pacing. EMI effects are temporary and do not usually cause permanent damage to the pacemaker device. The closer the pacemaker is to whatever is creating the electromagnetic field, the greater the effect, and the further away, the less of an effect is experienced. When patients are fitted with a pacemaker, they are given advice about which devices and situations to avoid (e.g., how to deal with airport security screening procedures).

Many resources are available online regarding safe use of pacemakers, including guidance provided by various manufacturers of pacemakers. For example, in the guidance documents provided by Boston Scientific, medical and dental devices that are considered safe to use with pacemakers (when used normally in accordance with their intended use) include dental drills and cleaning equipment, diagnostic x-rays, electrocardiogram (ECG), mammography, and ultrasound (BostonScientific, 2013). Similar clear guidance is provided by Medtronic, whose list of devices/procedures that pose "no known risk" to pacemakers (when the device is used as intended and is in good working order) includes acupuncture, bone density assessment, bone density ultrasound, dental drills, dental ultrasonic scalers/cleaners, diagnostic x-rays, ECG, hearing aids, laser surgery, mammography, positron emission tomography (PET scan), and sleep apnea machines (Medtronic, 2013). Similar to most companies, Medtronic further add: "Before undergoing any medical procedure, it is recommended that you advise your treating doctor or dentist that you have an implanted heart device and consult with your heart doctor to evaluate any possible associated risk." Similarly, St. Jude Medical indicate that there is "no known risk"

PATIENT ASSESSMENT

to pacemakers from dental drills and ultrasonic scalers (St. Jude Medical, 2013).

Despite the clear guidance from the manufacturers of pacemaker devices, the dental literature has tended to be much more cautious in approach, and this has doubtless stemmed from fears of causing harm following research that has suggested that ultrasonic instruments may produce EMI that could impair pacemaker function. Most of the research that identified a potential impact of ultrasonic instruments on pacemaker function was conducted using older models of pacemakers which, unlike modern devices, were not well shielded against possible sources of EMI. Indeed, a number of publications in dental journals in the 1970s and 1980s counseled against the use of ultrasonic instruments in patients with pacemakers (Adams et al., 1982; Griffiths, 1978; Rezai, 1977). In the late 1990s, in an *in vitro* study, inhibition of pacing from two brands of pacemakers was reported when a magnetostrictive ultrasonic scaler was placed in close proximity to the pacemakers (up to a distance of 15.0–37.5 cm, depending on the brand of the instrument) (Miller et al., 1998). In a similar study that had been conducted earlier, however, no interference with pacemaker function was recorded following the use of ultrasonic instruments (Luker, 1982). An American Academy of Periodontology (AAP) position paper published in 2000 recommended avoiding the use of ultrasonic instruments in patients with pacemakers (Drisko et al., 2000), though this paper was rescinded in 2007 (Journal of Periodontology, 2007). In 2010, an *in vitro* study reported interference with the activity of pacemakers when an ultrasonic scaler was operated in close proximity to the pacemakers (up to 23 cm), and also interference with an implantable cardioverter-defibrillator (ICD) (at 7 cm from the leads) (Roedig et al., 2010). However, the validity of these findings was subsequently disputed (specifically, it was asserted that the ultrasonic scaler interfered only with the telemetry of the pacemakers, and did not cause inhibition of pacing), and it also transpired that older pacemaker

models had been used in the research (Carlson, 2010; Crossley and Poole, 2010). In relation to ICD devices, an *in vitro* study identified that ultrasonic scalers failed to produce any interference with the device at the minimum distance of 2.5 cm utilized (Brand et al., 2007).

Review papers that have focused on this issue have tended to conclude that magnetostrictive ultrasonic scalers should be avoided in people with pacemakers, because of the theoretical risk of interfering with pacemaker function, and have also suggested that more research on this matter is indicated due to the better shielding of modern pacemaker units (Stoopler et al., 2011; Trenter and Walmsley, 2003). On the other hand, manufacturers of modern pacemakers state unequivocally in their guidance documents and on their websites that there is no known risk to pacemaker function posed by dental ultrasonic instruments (assuming that the ultrasonic scalers are in good working order, and properly grounded). Cardiologists seem to be similarly unconcerned – for example, in a review of causes of interference with implanted cardiac devices published in 2002, ultrasonic instruments (or even dentistry in general) were not even mentioned as a possible cause of problems (Pinski and Trohman, 2002).

How, then, should we manage the patient who requires RSD, but who also has a pacemaker? One option would be to only provide hand instrumentation, but this is contrary to modern concepts of effective periodontal management, in which the preference is to use ultrasonic instruments with a light-touch approach to disrupt the biofilm and minimize tooth damage. Indeed, it could be argued that by *not* providing ultrasonic RSD, the benefits of treatment would be limited, and this would compromise resolution of inflammation and healing potential in patients with pacemakers. In other words, the dental clinician must consider whether it would be in the patient's best interests to *withhold* the use of the ultrasonic instrument. It is also important to remember that the dentist is an autonomous primary care provider, who is, of all the healthcare providers, best trained and equipped with the necessary knowledge to make the correct treatment decisions about how to manage the oral health of his/her patients. In other words, decision-making on this issue remains the dentist's responsibility, and though information and advice may sometimes be sought from a medical colleague, the dentist remains responsible for considering the available evidence in the context of the patient's clinical needs and wishes, and then making a treatment decision collaboratively with the patient that is in the patient's best interests (Gary and Glick, 2012; Glick, 2011).

The apparently widely held viewpoint in dentistry contraindicating the use of ultrasonic scalers in patients with pacemakers is not substantiated by the available evidence. Cardiologists appear unconcerned on this matter, and pacemaker manufacturers clearly state that there is no known risk in their published guidance documents. To the best of the authors' knowledge, no instance of interference with pacemaker function has ever been reported in a patient undergoing ultrasonic instrumentation. There appear to be no compelling reasons to contraindicate the use of ultrasonic scalers in patients with pacemakers, and electively withholding their use in such patients may compromise outcomes of treatment. Taking all these factors into account, and consistent with the advice given by the pacemaker manufacturers, we consider that there is no particular concern with using magnetostrictive ultrasonic scalers in patients with modern pacemakers, and that they can and should be used if clinically indicated.

Vagus nerve stimulators

Vagus nerve stimulators are implanted devices used in both adult and pediatric patients primarily for the management of epilepsy that cannot be controlled by medications or other surgical methods. Vagus nerve stimulation with an implantable pulse generator is an effective

therapy for epilepsy, although the precise mechanism of action is unclear (Connor et al., 2012). The device is implanted below the left clavicle with the electrode positioned in the left vagus nerve, and is activated by the patient whenever they begin to feel the aura that can precede an epileptic seizure. A number of dental devices, including an ultrasonic scaler, have been tested to identify whether there is any interference with vagus nerve stimulator function. None of the tested devices (including the ultrasonic instrument) generated a magnetic field that was sufficient to influence pulse generator function, and it was concluded that ultrasonic scalers may be used in patients who have implanted vagus nerve stimulators without any adverse effects (Roberts, 2002). As with other implanted devices, it is important for the dental clinician to record the presence of a vagus nerve stimulator when obtaining the medical history, as well as ascertaining details of the aura symptoms that a patient may experience, and the responsibilities of the dental team in case of a seizure (Lisowska and Daly, 2012).

Pregnancy

A large number of studies have investigated the relationship between adverse pregnancy outcomes (low birth weight and/or preterm birth) and presence of maternal periodontitis. Two mechanisms have been purported to link adverse pregnancy outcomes and periodontitis. The first is that pregnant females who also have periodontitis may experience more frequent bacteremias, increasing the exposure of the fetal-placental unit to bacteria and their by-products, which could result in an inflammatory cascade leading to preterm birth. The second proposed mechanism is that inflammatory mediators produced locally in periodontitis enter the circulation, resulting in upregulated systemic inflammation and leading to preterm labor. A large number of studies have focused on whether treatment of maternal periodontal disease can reduce the risk of adverse pregnancy outcomes, but the largest and highest quality randomized controlled trials that have investigated this issue have consistently shown no beneficial effect of periodontal therapy on pregnancy outcomes (Chambrone et al., 2011; Michalowicz et al., 2013). This is understandable because targeting a single issue (i.e., periodontitis) will not address many of the other risk factors that are common to both periodontitis and adverse pregnancy outcomes, such as smoking, low socio-economic status, and diabetes. There appears to be no justification, therefore, for advocating that periodontal therapy is undertaken as a means by which to improve pregnancy outcomes (Michalowicz et al., 2013).

However, the large number of clinical studies that have been conducted to date have demonstrated that nonsurgical periodontal treatment in pregnant women is safe, whether undertaken using hand instruments and a root planing strategy, or whether undertaken using ultrasonic instruments and a RSD strategy. Furthermore, the large numbers of treatment studies in pregnant women that have been reported have confirmed that clinically significant improvements in periodontal status are achieved as a result of nonsurgical therapy. Pregnant females with periodontitis should, therefore, receive standard nonsurgical periodontal therapy with the goal of disrupting and reducing the bacterial biofilm and reducing periodontal inflammation (Sanz and Kornman, 2013). There is no evidence to suggest that dental (and periodontal treatment) is at all harmful to the pregnant woman or her developing fetus (Boggess, 2008). It is certainly the case that periodontal treatment is beneficial in its own right in pregnant females, many of whom may experience pregnancy gingivitis, and clinicians should provide the necessary therapy to improve oral hygiene and minimize gingival and periodontal inflammation (Armitage, 2013). Potentially, ultrasonic RSD may confer an advantage when treating a pregnant patient who also has periodontitis, in that shorter appointment times may be achievable (compared to using hand instruments), which may make the treatment

more tolerable, particularly in the later stages of pregnancy.

Pediatric patients

Assessment of periodontal status is equally important in children as it is in adults, and periodontal screening should be performed routinely in children. Children can often present with gingivitis, but chronic periodontitis, aggressive periodontitis and acute periodontal conditions may also be identified (Clerehugh and Tugnait, 2001). Periodontal treatment should be provided as clinically indicated, and plaque control programs have been shown to be effective in preventing gingivitis in children (Ashley and Sainsbury, 1981; Badersten et al., 1975). RSD is indicated in children with evidence of periodontitis (both chronic periodontitis and aggressive periodontitis), including children in both the primary or mixed dentition stages. Ultrasonic instruments are routinely used safely in children, but the clinician needs to be aware that the enamel is significantly thinner in deciduous teeth than it is in permanent adult teeth (Grine, 2005). For this reason, to avoid sensitivity and possible pulpitis resulting from thermal trauma, the usual principles of ultrasonic usage should be maintained, such as adequate water irrigation, keeping the tip moving, light pressure, and using reduced power settings on the ultrasonic device.

REFERENCES

Adams D, Fulford N, Beechy J, MacCarthy J, Stephens M. The cardiac pacemaker and ultrasonic scalers. *Br Dent J* 1982; 152: 171–3.

Arabaci T, Cicek Y, Ozgoz M, Canakci V, Canakci CF, Eltas A. The comparison of the effects of three types of piezoelectric ultrasonic tips and air polishing system on the filling materials: an in vitro study. *Int J Dent Hyg* 2007; 5: 205–10.

Armitage GC. Bi-directional relationship between pregnancy and periodontal disease. *Periodontol 2000* 2013; 61: 160–76.

Ashley FP, Sainsbury RH. The effect of a school-based plaque control programme on caries and gingivitis. A 3-year study in 11 to 14-year-old girls. *Br Dent J* 1981; 150: 41–5.

Badersten A, Egelberg J, Koch G. Effect of monthly prophylaxis on caries and gingivitis in schoolchildren. *Community Dent Oral Epidemiol* 1975; 3: 1–4.

Badersten A, Nilveus RE, Egelberg JH. Effect of nonsurgical periodontal therapy. I. Moderately advanced periodontitis. *J Clin Periodontol* 1981; 8: 57–72.

Badersten A, Nilveus RE, Egelberg JH. Effect of nonsurgical periodontal therapy. II. Severely advanced periodontitis. *J Clin Periodontol* 1984; 11: 63–76.

Badersten A, Nilveus RE, Egelberg JH. Effect of nonsurgical periodontal therapy. IV. Operator variability. *J Clin Periodontol* 1985; 12: 190–200.

Bjornson EJ, Collins DE, Engler WO. Surface alteration of composite resins after curette, ultrasonic, and sonic instrumentation: an in vitro study. *Quintessence Int* 1990; 21: 381–9.

Boggess KA. Maternal oral health in pregnancy. *Obstet Gynecol* 2008; 111: 976–86.

Booker BW, Loughlin DM. A morphologic study of the mesial root surface of the adolescent maxillary first bicuspid. *J Periodontol* 1985; 56: 666–70.

BostonScientific. At Home – Work – Play. Living in a world with EMI (Electromagnetic Interference) [Internet]. 2013 (updated January 2013; cited 7 June 2013). Available at http://www.bostonscientific.com/lifebeat-online/resources/patient-electromagnetic-interference.html?

Bower RC. Furcation morphology relative to periodontal treatment. Furcation entrance architecture. *J Periodontol* 1979a; 50: 23–7.

Bower RC. Furcation morphology relative to periodontal treatment. Furcation root surface anatomy. *J Periodontol* 1979b; 50: 366–74.

Brand HS, Entjes ML, Nieuw Amerongen AV, van der Hoeff EV, Schrama TA. Interference of electrical dental equipment with implantable cardioverter-defibrillators. *Br Dent J* 2007; 203: 577–9.

Burch JG, Hulen S. A study of the presence of accessory foramina and the topography of molar furcations. *Oral Surg Oral Med Oral Pathol* 1974; 38: 451–5.

Carlson BK. Pacemakers and dental devices. *J Am Dent Assoc* 2010; 141: 1052–3.

Cattabriga M, Pedrazzoli V, Wilson TG Jr. The conservative approach in the treatment of furcation lesions. *Periodontol 2000* 2000; 22: 133–53.

Chambrone L, Pannuti CM, Guglielmetti MR, Chambrone LA. Evidence grade associating periodontitis with preterm birth and/or low birth weight: II: a systematic review of randomized trials evaluating the effects of periodontal treatment. *J Clin Periodontol* 2011; 38: 902–14.

Chapple ILC. Periodontal disease diagnosis: current status and future developments. *J Dent* 1997; 25: 3–15.

Claffey N, Nylund K, Kiger R, Garrett S, Egelberg J. Diagnostic predictability of scores of plaque, bleeding, suppuration and probing depth for probing attachment loss. 3 1/2 years of observation following initial periodontal therapy. *J Clin Periodontol* 1990; 17: 108–14.

Clerehugh V, Tugnait A. Diagnosis and management of periodontal diseases in children and adolescents. *Periodontol 2000* 2001; 26: 146–68.

Cobb CM. Non-surgical pocket therapy: mechanical. *Ann Periodontol* 1996; 1: 443–90.

Cobb CM. Clinical significance of non-surgical periodontal therapy: an evidence-based perspective of scaling and root planing. *J Clin Periodontol* 2002; 29 (Suppl. 2): 6–16.

Connor DE Jr., Nixon M, Nanda A, Guthikonda B. Vagal nerve stimulation for the treatment of medically refractory epilepsy: a review of the current literature. *Neurosurg Focus* 2012; 32: E12.

Crossley GH, Poole JE. More about pacemakers. *J Am Dent Assoc* 2010; 141: 1053.

Del Peloso Ribeiro E, Bittencourt S, Nociti FH Jr., Sallum EA, Sallum AW, Casati MZ. Comparative study of ultrasonic instrumentation for the non-surgical treatment of interproximal and non-interproximal furcation involvements. *J Periodontol* 2007; 78: 224–30.

dos Santos KM, Pinto SC, Pochapski MT, Wambier DS, Pilatti GL, Santos FA. Molar furcation entrance and its relation to the width of curette blades used in periodontal mechanical therapy. *Int J Dent Hyg* 2009; 7: 263–9.

Drisko CL, Cochran DL, Blieden T, Bouwsma OJ, Cohen RE, Damoulis P, Fine JB, Greenstein G, Hinrichs J, Somerman MJ, Iacono V, Genco RJ. Position paper: sonic and ultrasonic scalers in periodontics. Research, Science and Therapy Committee of the American Academy of Periodontology. *J Periodontol* 2000; 71: 1792–801

Flemmig TF, Petersilka GJ, Mehl A, Hickel R, Klaiber B. The effect of working parameters on root substance removal using a piezoelectric ultrasonic scaler in vitro. *J Clin Periodontol* 1998; 25: 158–63.

PATIENT ASSESSMENT

Gary CJ, Glick M. Medical clearance: an issue of professional autonomy, not a crutch. *J Am Dent Assoc* 2012; 143: 1180–1.

Gher ME, Vernino AR. Root morphology - clinical significance in pathogenesis and treatment of periodontal disease. *J Am Dent Assoc* 1980; 101: 627–33.

Glick M. Clinical judgment: a requirement for professional identity. *J Am Dent Assoc* 2011; 142: 1333–4.

Glickman I (1953) The treatment of bifurcation and trifurcation involvement. In: *Clinical Periodontology*, pp. 794–803. Philadelphia: WB Saunders.

Gorfil C, Nordenberg D, Liberman R, Ben-Amar A. The effect of ultrasonic cleaning and air polishing on the marginal integrity of radicular amalgam and composite resin restorations. An in vitro study. *J Clin Periodontol* 1989; 16: 137–9.

Griffiths PV. The management of the pacemaker wearer during dental hygiene treatment. *Dent Hyg* 1978; 52: 573–6.

Grine FE. Enamel thickness of deciduous and permanent molars in modern Homo sapiens. *Am J Phys Anthropol* 2005; 126: 14–31.

Hamp SE, Nyman S, Lindhe J. Periodontal treatment of multi-rooted teeth. Results after 5 years. *J Clin Periodontol* 1975; 2: 126–35.

Hefti AF. Periodontal probing. *Crit Rev Oral Biol Med* 1997; 8: 336–56.

Hou GL, Chen SF, Wu YM, Tsai CC. The topography of the furcation entrance in Chinese molars: furcation entrance dimensions. *J Clin Periodontol* 1994; 21: 451–6.

Journal of Periodontology. Position paper update. *J Periodontol* 2007; 78: 1476.

Lai YL, Lin YC, Chang CS, Lee SY. Effects of sonic and ultrasonic scaling on the surface roughness of tooth-colored restorative materials for cervical lesions. *Oper Dent* 2007; 32: 273–8.

Lang NP, Adler R, Joss A, Nyman S. Absence of bleeding on probing. An indicator of periodontal stability. *J Clin Periodontol* 1990; 17: 714–21.

Lang NP, Joss A, Orsanic T, Gusberti FA, Siegrist BE. Bleeding on probing. A predictor for the progression of periodontal disease? *J Clin Periodontol* 1986; 13: 590–6.

Leon LE, Vogel RI. A comparison of the effectiveness of hand scaling and ultrasonic debridement in furcations as evaluated by differential dark-field microscopy. *J Periodontol* 1987; 58: 86–94.

Lindhe J, Okamoto H, Yoneyama T, Haffajee A, Socransky SS. Longitudinal changes in periodontal disease in untreated subjects. *J Clin Periodontol* 1989; 16: 662–70.

Lindhe J, Socransky SS, Nyman S, Haffajee AD, Westfelt E. "Critical probing depths" in periodontal therapy. *J Clin Periodontol* 1982; 9: 323–36.

Lisowska P, Daly B. Vagus nerve stimulation therapy (VNST) in epilepsy - implications for dental practice. *Br Dent J* 2012; 212: 69–72.

Luker J. The pacemaker patient in the dental surgery. *J Dent* 1982; 10: 326–32.

Matia JI, Bissada NF, Maybury JE, Ricchetti P. Efficiency of scaling of the molar furcation area with and without surgical access. *Int J Periodontics Restorative Dent* 1986; 6: 24–35.

Medtronic. More help for heart device patients. Electromagnetic Compatibility Guide [Internet]. 2013 (cited 7 June 2013). Available at http://www.medtronic.com/rhythms/downloads/UC200602918EN.pdf.

Michalowicz BS, Gustafsson A, Thumbigere-Math V, Buhlin K. The effects of periodontal treatment on pregnancy outcomes. *J Clin Periodontol* 2013; 40 Suppl 14: S195–208.

Miller CS, Leonelli FM, Latham E. Selective interference with pacemaker activity by electrical dental devices. *Oral Surg Oral Med Oral Pathol Oral Radiol Endodont* 1998; 85: 33–6.

Oda S, Ishikawa I. In vitro effectiveness of a newly-designed ultrasonic scaler tip for furcation areas. *J Periodontol* 1989; 60: 634–9.

Osborn JB, Stoltenberg JL, Huso BA, Aeppli DM, Pihlstrom BL. Comparison of measurement variability in subjects with moderate periodontitis using a conventional and constant force periodontal probe. *J Periodontol* 1992; 63: 283–9.

Pihlstrom BL, McHugh R, Oliphant T, Ortiz-Campos C. Comparison of surgical and nonsurgical treatment of periodontal disease. A review of current studies and additional results after 6 1/2 years. *J Clin Periodontol* 1983; 10: 524–41.

Pinski SL, Trohman RG. Interference in implanted cardiac devices, part II. *Pacing Clin Electrophysiol* 2002; 25: 1496–509.

Preshaw PM, Alba AL, Herrera D, Jepsen S, Konstantinidis A, Makrilakis K, Taylor R. Periodontitis and diabetes: a two-way relationship. *Diabetologia* 2012; 55: 21–31.

Rezai FR. Dental treatment of patient with a cardiac pacemaker. Review of the literature. *Oral Surg Oral Med Oral Pathol* 1977; 44: 662–5.

PATIENT ASSESSMENT

Roberts HW. The effect of electrical dental equipment on a vagus nerve stimulator's function. *J Am Dent Assoc* 2002; 133: 1657–64.

Roedig JJ, Shah J, Elayi CS, Miller CS. Interference of cardiac pacemaker and implantable cardioverter-defibrillator activity during electronic dental device use. *J Am Dent Assoc* 2010; 141: 521–6.

Sanz M, Kornman K. Periodontitis and adverse pregnancy outcomes: consensus report of the Joint EFP/AAP Workshop on Periodontitis and Systemic Diseases. *J Clin Periodontol* 2013; 40 Suppl 14: S164–9.

Schatzle M, Loe H, Burgin W, Anerud A, Boysen H, Lang NP. Clinical course of chronic periodontitis. I. Role of gingivitis. *J Clin Periodontol* 2003; 30: 887–901.

Scott JB, Steed-Veilands AM, Yukna RA. Improved efficacy of calculus removal in furcations using ultrasonic diamond-coated inserts. *Int J Periodontics Restorative Dent* 1999; 19: 355–61.

St. Jude Medical. Electromagnetic Interference (EMI) in the home or medical environment [Internet]. 2013 (updated 25 April 2011; cited 10 June 2013). Available at http://health.sjm.com /heart-failure-answers/daily-life/everyday-concerns-with-an-implantable-device/electromagnetic-interference-emi.

Stoopler ET, Sia YW, Kuperstein AS. Does ultrasonic dental equipment affect cardiovascular implantable electronic devices? *J Dent Can Assoc* 2011; 77: b113.

Sugaya T, Kawanami M, Kato H. Accessibility of an ultrasonic furcation tip to furcation areas of mandibular first and second molars. *J Int Acad Periodontol* 2002; 4: 132–7.

Takacs VJ, Lie T, Perala DG, Adams DF. Efficacy of 5 machining instruments in scaling of molar furcations. *J Periodontol* 1993; 64: 228–36.

Trenter SC, Walmsley AD. Ultrasonic dental scaler: associated hazards. *J Clin Periodontol* 2003; 30: 95–101.

Walmsley AD, Lumley PJ, Blunt L, Spence D. Surface integrity of composite inlays following ultrasonic vibration. *Am J Dent* 1997; 10: 102–6.

PATIENT ASSESSMENT

Chapter 6

Ultrasonic instrumentation technique

CHAPTER OBJECTIVES

On completion of this chapter, the student will be able to:

1. Demonstrate the basic principles of ultrasonic instrumentation technique.

2. Explain the relationship between each instrumentation technique variable and the removal of deposits and root substance.

3. Identify infection control procedures, which will minimize cross-contamination by the aerosol generated during ultrasonic instrumentation.

4. Justify the staged approach to ultrasonic periodontal instrumentation.

Manual and ultrasonic instrumentation share the common objective of thorough disruption and removal of biofilm and calculus deposits without over-instrumentation of the root surface; however, the mechanisms by which each instrumentation method achieves this objective significantly differ, are inherent to the design of each instrument, and influence the instrumentation technique utilized.

Hand scaling instruments are designed to mechanically break the bond between the deposit and the tooth at the tooth–deposit interface by manually stroking a bladed cutting edge across the tooth surface (Lea and Walmsley, 2009). As presented in Chapter 3, ultrasonic scaling instruments are designed to ablate and disrupt deposits by vibratory and biophysical forces produced by a blunt metal tip oscillating at a high frequency (Walmsley et al., 1984; Khambay and Walmsley, 1999).

While ultrasonic and manual instrumentation methods are equally effective in removing deposits and improving and maintaining periodontal health as measured by reduction in clinical parameters (BOP, PD, CAL) (Chapter 2), ultrasonic instrumentation is less damaging to the root surface than hand instrumentation (Ritz et al., 1991; Dragoo, 1992; Jacobson et al., 1994; Busslinger et al., 2001; Schmidlin et al., 2001; Kawashima et al., 2007). However, the amount of root substance lost during ultrasonic instrumentation is technique-dependent (Box 6.1).

Box 6.1: Key point

Both the effectiveness of deposit removal and the amount of root surface lost during ultrasonic instrumentation are *technique-dependent*!

Ultrasonic Periodontal Debridement: Theory and Technique, First Edition. Marie D. George, Timothy G. Donley and Philip M. Preshaw.
© 2014 John Wiley & Sons, Inc. Published 2014 by John Wiley & Sons, Inc.

In order to accomplish the objectives of periodontal debridement by means of ultrasonic mechanisms of action, it is prudent for the clinician to have a solid understanding of the ultrasonic instrumentation technique and the variables that influence both deposit removal and root substance loss.

ULTRASONIC INSTRUMENTATION: PRINCIPLES OF TECHNIQUE

A significant error commonly made during ultrasonic debridement is the implementation of principles of manual instrumentation, with clinicians inappropriately utilizing the ultrasonic instrument as a "hand scaler with power." Such misapplication of the ultrasonic scaling instrument is largely due to a lack of instructional resources specific to ultrasonic instrumentation theory and technique compounded by training curricula historically grounded in hand (manual) instrumentation.

The *principles of technique* for ultrasonic instrumentation are summarized and differentiated from the principles of technique for manual instrumentation in Table 6.1.

Adaptation

The stroke pattern produced by the oscillating ultrasonic tip influences instrumentation technique, specifically the adaptation of the tip to the tooth.

Contrary to popular belief, both piezoelectric and magnetostrictive instruments produce an elliptical stroke pattern (Chapter 3), which allows debridement to be accomplished by adapting any surface of the oscillating tip to the tooth. The ability to utilize any surface of the tip (back, face, or lateral surfaces) facilitates a greater degree of contact between the active area and treatment surface, and thus, a more efficient and predictable debridement. A greater degree of contact results when the shape of the active tip conforms to the anatomy of the treatment surface (Figure 6.1).

Achieving a greater degree of contact is dependent upon not just the shape of the tip utilized, but more precisely, which surface of the tip is adapted and the manner in which the surface is adapted. Preferably, the surface of the tip that best conforms to the anatomy of the treatment surface should be utilized; however, at some treatment sites, this will not be possible.

Table 6.1 Comparison of principles: techniques of periodontal instrumentation

Principle	Ultrasonic instrumentation	Hand instrumentation
Adaptation	Adapt any surface of the active tip • Vertical orientation • Horizontal orientation (interproximal surfaces only)	Adapt lateral surface of toe/tip • Oblique orientation
Angulation	0–15° to tooth surface	45–90° to tooth surface
Lateral pressure	Light pressure applied to maintain contact with tooth	Moderate pressure applied to engage cutting edge
Working Stroke	Constant and varied in direction	Intermittent and apico-coronal in direction
Insertion	At gingival margin or outer edge of deposit	Below deposit
Grasp	Light standard pen	Firm modified pen
Fulcrum	Established at a distance from treatment site for stabilization	Established in immediate treatment area to leverage working stroke

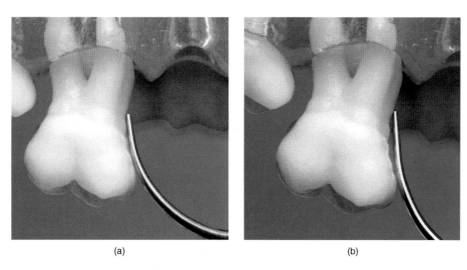

(a)	(b)

Figure 6.1 Adaptation of the back of a tip to the mesial concavity of tooth #3 (FDI 16). The convex arc of the curved tip (a) conforms to the concave anatomy of the tooth surface, whereas adaptation of a straight tip (b) lacks conformity, leaving a gap between the tip and tooth surface

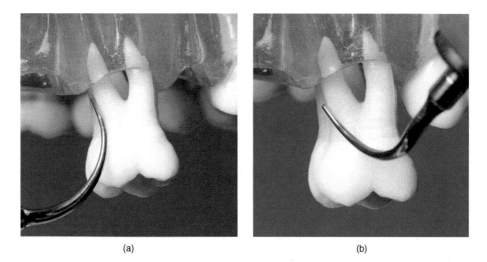

(a)	(b)

Figure 6.2 In a distal concavity, (a) adaptation of the convex back of the tip is ideal, but impossible to achieve; as an alternative, (b) the lateral surface of the tip is adapted

Alternatively then, the tip surface most readily available to the treatment surface can and should be used (Figure 6.2).

The preferred surface of the ultrasonic tip may be adapted to the tooth using several orientations: vertical (parallel) adaptation, horizontal (perpendicular) adaptation, and traditional oblique adaptation. Indications for use of each of these orientations are designated in Table 6.2.

A. Vertical (parallel) adaptation

Vertical adaptation positions the active area of the ultrasonic tip parallel to the long

Table 6.2 Ultrasonic instrumentation adaptation techniques

Image	Adaptation technique	Description	Indication for use
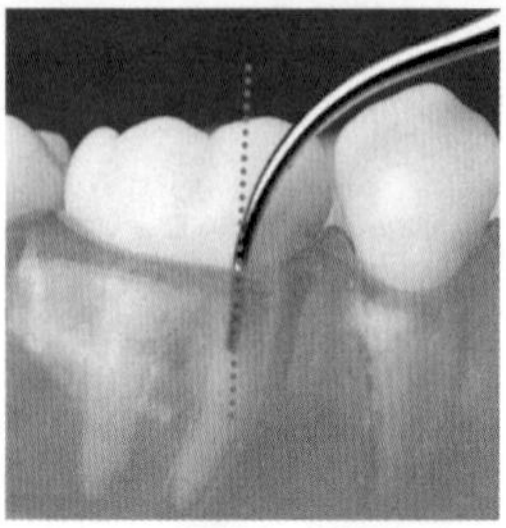	**Vertical (Parallel)**	Active area of tip is parallel to long axis of tooth, with point of tip directed apically, toward base of the pocket	Instrumentation of all subgingival and supragingival surfaces (excluding interproximal spaces) using any surface of the tip
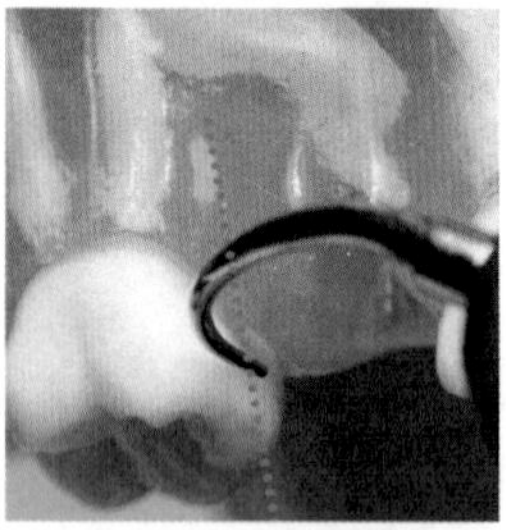	**Horizontal (Perpendicular)**	Active area of tip is perpendicular to the long axis of the tooth	Instrumentation of interproximal space using back or face of the tip
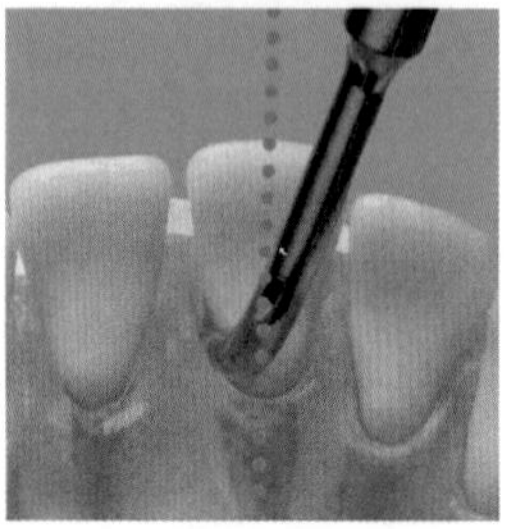	**Oblique**	Active area of a lateral surface is oblique to the long axis of the tooth	Manual instrumentation; not recommended by authors for ultrasonic instrumentation

axis of the tooth, with the point of the tip directed toward the base of the pocket (Figure 6.3). This is the same orientation used during periodontal probing (Figure 6.4).

Vertical adaptation is the primary and preferred approach to be used during ultrasonic debridement for several reasons:

– As accomplished during periodontal probing, vertical orientation facilitates the most direct access to the base of deeper pockets, increasing the predictability of the active area of the tip reaching the full depth of the treatment site (Figure 6.5).

– The extent of biofilm removed by cavitation and microstreaming may be increased with vertical adaptation to the tooth. Walmsley et al (1988) demonstrated that vertical adaptation of the tip resulted in an eightfold increase in biofilm removal, compared to a sixfold increase in biofilm removal when the tip was adapted in the more traditional oblique orientation (Figures 6.6a,b).

– Vertical orientation favors easy adaptation of ANY surface of the tip to any surface of the tooth. From this orientation, the

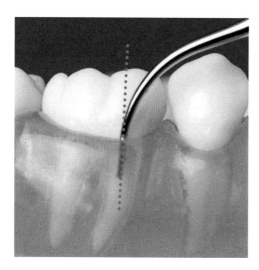

Figure 6.3 Vertical adaptation of the tip. Tip is positioned parallel to the long axis of the tooth with point directed toward the base of the pocket

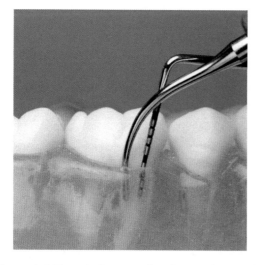

Figure 6.4 Vertical adaptation of an ultrasonic tip is similar to the adaptation of periodontal probe

clinician can readily adapt the preferred tip surface to the tooth with minimal repositioning required (Figure 6.7).

– On concave and convex tooth surfaces, positioning the tip parallel to the surface yields contact of a greater portion of the active tip area (2–3 mm vs 1–2 mm if positioned obliquely), maximizing the

surface area debrided with each stroke and requiring fewer strokes per treatment surface (Figure 6.8).

B. Horizontal (perpendicular) adaptation

Horizontal adaptation, which may also be described as "perpendicular" adaptation, is used primarily for instrumentation in the interproximal space (Figure 6.9). Horizontal adaptation positions the active area of the tip perpendicular, or in a horizontal orientation, to the long axis of the tooth, facilitating use of the BACK and FACE of the active tip.

Horizontal adaptation to the interproximal surfaces affords the clinician an easier and more ergonomic transition to and from the primary position of vertical adaptation than does traditional oblique adaptation. This transition is fully described in Chapter 7, General Principles of Instrumentation Sequencing.

C. Oblique adaptation

Oblique adaptation positions the active area of the LATERAL surface of the tip in an oblique orientation to the long axis of the tooth (Figure 6.10). This is the same orientation used with bladed instruments, such as curettes and sickle scalers.

Use of oblique adaptation is one of the common misapplications of the ultrasonic instrument alluded to at the beginning of this chapter. Oblique adaptation is necessary during manual instrumentation in order to keep the cutting edge, located on a lateral surface of the curette or sickle, in contact with the tooth and in a position that enables the clinician to stroke the cutting edge in a direction that will break the bond between the deposit and the tooth. In other words, oblique adaptation is inherent to the mechanism of removal for which hand instruments are designed.

As ultrasonic instruments utilize a very different mechanism of deposit removal, oblique

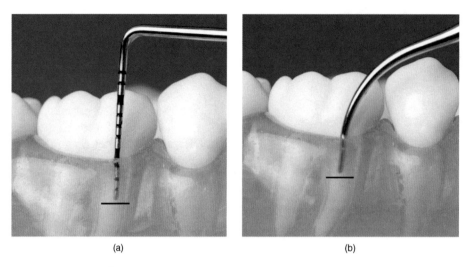

(a)   (b)

Figure 6.5 Vertical adaptation facilitates direct access to the base of the pocket during (a) periodontal probing and (b) ultrasonic instrumentation

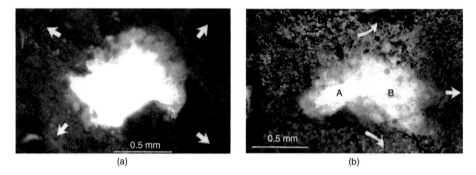

(a)   (b)

Figure 6.6 Extent of plaque removal by tip and cavitational activity resulting from (a) vertical adaptation of the tip compared to (b) oblique adaptation of the tip. The direction of water flow is indicated by arrows. (*Source*: Walmsley et al., 1988. Reproduced with permission of John Wiley & Sons, Inc.)

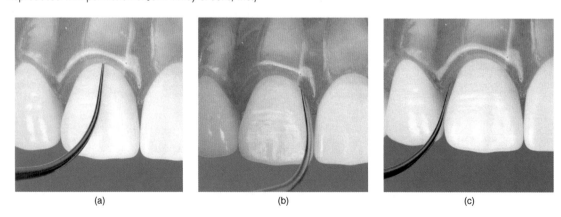

(a)   (b)   (c)

Figure 6.7 From vertical adaptation, the tip can be readily adapted to all tooth surfaces, (a) facial or lingual, (b) mesial, and (c) distal, without changing fulcrum or operator position

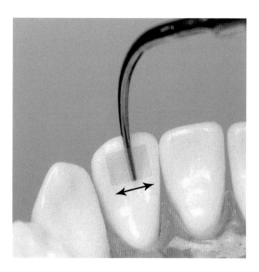

Figure 6.8 On a concave surface, vertical adaptation of the tip allows a greater portion of the active area to contact the tooth, increasing the surface area debrided (shaded area) with each stroke; arrow indicates direction of working stroke

adaptation is neither indicated nor recommended by these authors, as it imposes several limitations to implementing an effective and efficient debridement:

- Oblique adaptation limits the clinician to utilizing a lateral surface of the tip.

  - Depending on tip design, the lateral surface may not be the surface that best conforms to the anatomy of the treatment site, thereby risking inadequate contact for thorough biofilm debridement.

  - The lateral surface may not be readily available to the treatment site, thereby requiring more frequent changes in operator position in order to adapt it, as is necessary when performing manual instrumentation.

- Oblique orientation of the tip may result in less biofilm being removed by cavitation and microstreaming compared to vertical orientation (sixfold vs eightfold), as illustrated previously in Figure 6.6 (Walmsley et al., 1988).

- Oblique orientation may hinder access of the active area to the base of deeper pockets, lessening the predictability of thorough debridement (Figure 6.11).

- Oblique adaptation of the lateral surface limits contact of the active area to the terminal 1–2 mm of the tip on any given surface, minimizing the surface area debrided with each stroke and requiring more strokes per treatment surface (Figure 6.12).

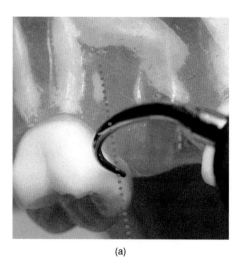

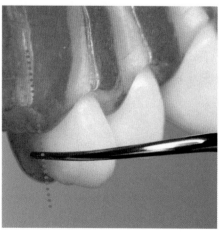

(a)   (b)

Figure 6.9 Horizontal adaptation of the tip. Tip position is perpendicular to the long axis of the tooth and facilitates use of (a) the back and (b) the face of the tip on interproximal coronal surfaces

ULTRASONIC INSTRUMENTATION TECHNIQUE

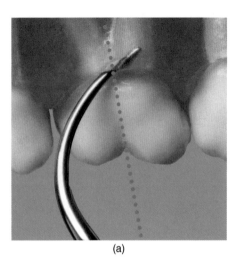
(a)

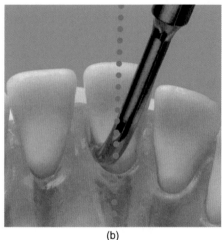
(b)

Figure 6.10 (a,b) Oblique adaptation of the tip. Tip position is oblique to the long axis of the tooth to facilitate adaptation of a lateral surface to the tooth

ULTRASONIC INSTRUMENTATION TECHNIQUE

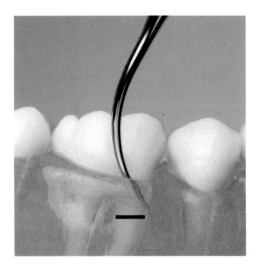

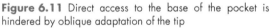

Figure 6.11 Direct access to the base of the pocket is hindered by oblique adaptation of the tip

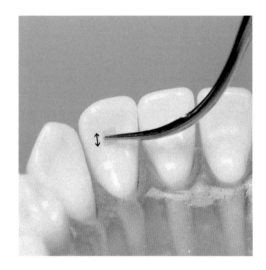

Figure 6.12 On a concave surface, oblique adaptation of the tip limits contact to the terminal 1–2 mm, minimizing the surface area debrided (shaded area) with each stroke; arrow indicates direction of working stroke

Angulation

Angulation of the active area of the oscillating tip to the tooth surface being treated should be maintained between *0 and 15 degrees*: as close to 0° as possible, but never exceeding 15° (Figure 6.13). By comparison, this is similar to the degree of angulation maintained during periodontal probing, and significantly less than the 45–90° cutting edge-to-tooth angulation (Nield-Gehrig, 2008) needed to accomplish manual scaling.

Increasing (opening) this tip-tooth angulation beyond the recommended 0–15° increases the amount of root substance lost during sonic and ultrasonic instrumentation.

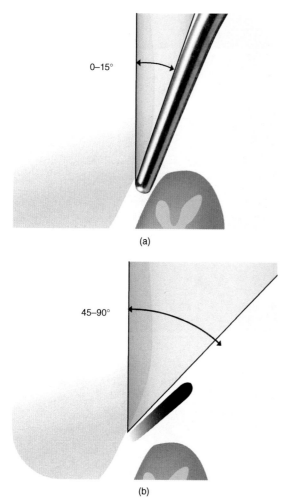

0–15°

(a)

45–90°

(b)

Figure 6.13 Angulation of the active area of the ultrasonic tip to the tooth surface is 0–15° (a), as compared to the 45–90° (b) angulation needed for manual instrumentation

Flemmig et al. (1997, 1998a,b) demonstrated a positive correlation between the amount of root surface lost and an increase in tip-tooth angulation. Using magnetostrictive technology (Flemmig et al., 1998b), as angulation of the tip increased from 0° to 45° to 90° to the tooth, so too did the depth of the root surface defect, regardless of power setting or lateral force (Figure 6.14). However, a different pattern of root surface loss was found when piezoelectric technology was evaluated. Using piezoelectric

technology (Flemmig et al., 1998a), significantly greater root surface loss occurred at the 45° angulation than at the 90° angulation (Figure 6.15).

At that time, the authors concluded that piezoelectric instruments are more technique sensitive in regard to tip angulation and alteration of the root surface than magnetostrictive instruments. In light of the findings of several subsequently published studies, which demonstrated that tip shape is more influential than type of generator on scaling performance (Lea et al., 2009a) and amount of root substance loss (Jepsen et al., 2004; Lea et al., 2009b) (see Chapters 3 and 4), it is likely that the differences between magnetostrictive and piezoelectric units observed by Flemmig et al. in regard to tip angulation and root surface alteration are also due to the differences in the tip shape used with each generator, not the type of generator, with the broad/flat (curette-like) tip used on the piezoelectric unit (Figure 6.16a) being more aggressive and angulation sensitive than the cylindrical (probe-like) tip used with the magnetostrictive unit (Figure 6.16b).

Lateral pressure

The tip is described as oscillating under *load* when it is adapted to the tooth surface, whereas the term *unloaded* refers to the tip oscillating freely in air. The degree of lateral pressure applied to adapt the tip is typically measured in Newtons (N), the standard unit of measurement of force.

The amount of lateral pressure to apply to the oscillating tip varies according to the type of deposit to be removed, ranging between 0.5 N and 2.0 N (Figure 6.17). Forces below this range (<0.5 N) may inhibit the clinician's ability to maintain continuous adaptation of the tip to the tooth. Forces above this range (>2 N) affect the efficiency of deposit removal and the amount of root surface damage.

By comparison, this is significantly less than the amount of lateral force applied during manual instrumentation, which has been demonstrated

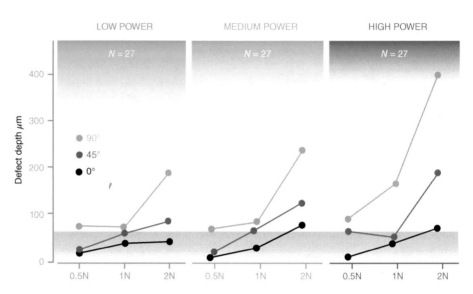

Figure 6.14 Effect of combinations of lateral force and tip angulation at different power settings on root surface defect depth after 40 seconds of instrumentation time using a magnetostrictive scaler. (*Source*: Flemmig et al., 1998b. Adapted with permission of the American Academy of Periodontology)

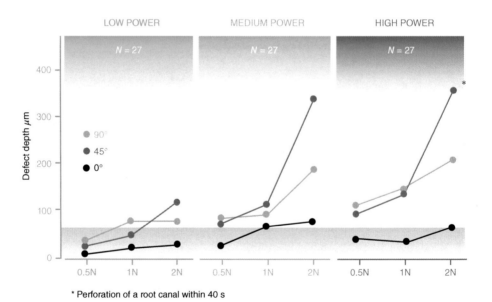

* Perforation of a root canal within 40 s

Figure 6.15 Effect of combinations of lateral forces and tip angulation at different power settings on root surface defect depth after 40 seconds of instrumentation time using a piezoelectric scaler. (*Source*: Flemmig et al., 1998a. Adapted with permission of John Wiley & Sons)

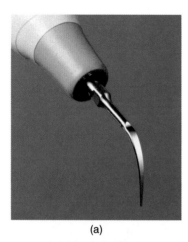

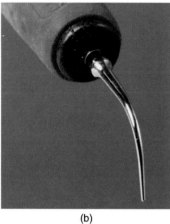

(a)

(b)

Figure 6.16 Tip designs identical or comparable to those used in the cited studies. Compare the (a) broad and flat (curette-like) design used with the piezoelectric scaling units to the (b) slim and cylindrical (probe-like) design used with the magnetostrictive scaling units

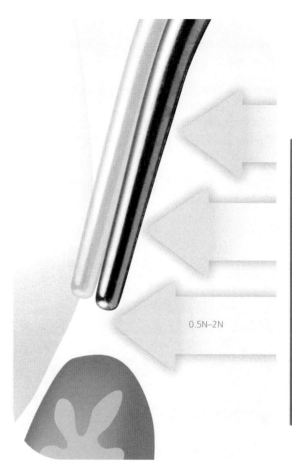

0.5N–2N

Figure 6.17 Range of lateral pressure applied during ultrasonic instrumentation

to range between 1.01 and 15.73 N, with a mean of 5.70 N applied by dentists and a mean of 5.38 N applied by dental hygienists (Zappa et al., 1991).

Influence of lateral pressure on deposit removal

When an oscillating tip contacts the tooth, there is a general tendency for displacement amplitude to decrease (or dampen) initially, but not continuously as lateral force increases up to 1.0 N

(Lea et al., 2003b; Trenter et al., 2003; Walmsley et al., 2013). Slim diameter tips appear to be more susceptible to dampening under load than wider diameter tips (Lea et al., 2003b; Trenter et al., 2003).

It has been previously established that the amount of cavitational activity is greater with wider diameter tips, increases with greater displacement amplitudes, and primarily occurs beyond the active area of the tip, at a vibration antinode (see Chapter 3). If application of lateral pressure constrains, or reduces, the displacement amplitude, it is rational to expect a concurrent reduction in cavitational activity.

ULTRASONIC INSTRUMENTATION TECHNIQUE

Instead, Walmsley et al. (2012) demonstrated that loading at forces of 1 N and 2 N increased the production of cavitation at low power settings and changed the distribution of the cavitational activity, from primarily at the antinode to more occurring at the clinically useful active area of the tip, especially with slim diameter tips (Figure 6.18).

These findings have clinical significance, as lower power settings and slimmer diameter tips are indicated to accomplish biofilm debridement

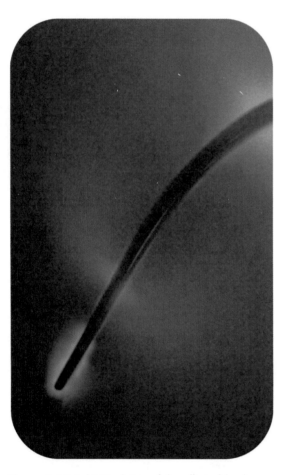

Figure 6.18 (a,b) Simulation of the effect of loading on an ultrasonic scaling tip at power 10/10. Application of load shifts the distribution of cavitation, resulting in increased cavitational activity at the active area of the tip (*Source*: Felver et al., 2009. Modified with permission from Elsevier)

without over-instrumentation of the root surface. Abiding by these working parameters, cavitation can be optimized to enhance the removal of biofilm with the application of lateral forces equivalent to 1 or 2 N.

Influence of lateral pressure on the root surface

Regarding the influence of lateral force on alteration of the root surface, increases in lateral force generally result in an increase in the amount of root surface lost. Lateral forces assessed include 0.3 N (Jepsen et al., 2004), 0.5 N (Flemmig et al., 1998a,b), 0.7 N (Jepsen et al., 2004), 1 N and 2 N (Flemmig et al., 1998a,b; Lea et al., 2009b). At any given power setting (Flemmig et al., 1998a,b; Jepsen et al., 2004; Lea et al., 2009b) or angulation (Flemmig et al., 1998a,b), an increase in lateral force correlates to an increase in the volume and depth of the root surface defect.

It is imperative for the clinician to understand that the working parameters of lateral force, tip angulation, and power setting, when combined, have additive effects on the amount of root surface lost (Flemmig et al., 1998a,b; Jepsen et al., 2004; Lea et al., 2009b), with lateral force and tip angulation having greater impact on root surface damage than power setting (Flemmig et al., 1998a,b). The synergistic effects of lateral force, tip angulation, and power setting on the amount of root substance removed are illustrated in Figures 6.19 and 6.20. Combinations of working parameters that limit root surface damage to the clinically acceptable depth of less than 50 μm per year should be utilized (Flemmig et al., 1998a,b).

As with tip angulation, Flemmig et al. (1998a) found the piezoelectric scaling unit to be more technique sensitive regarding lateral pressure than the magnetostrictive scaler (1998b), recommending that no more than 0.5 N lateral pressure be applied when using a piezoelectric generator, while up to 2 N of lateral force could be applied using a magnetostrictive generator without excessive root surface damage, assuming

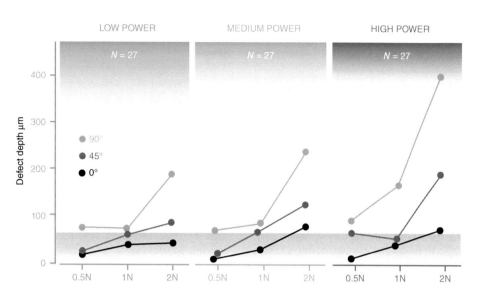

Figure 6.19 Effect of all combinations of lateral force and tip angulation at different power settings on defect depth after 40 seconds of instrumentation using a magnetostrictive scaler. The shaded area indicates combinations of working parameters resulting in a clinically acceptable defect depth of less than 50 μm (*Source*: Flemmig et al., 1998b. Adapted with permission of the American Academy of Periodontology)

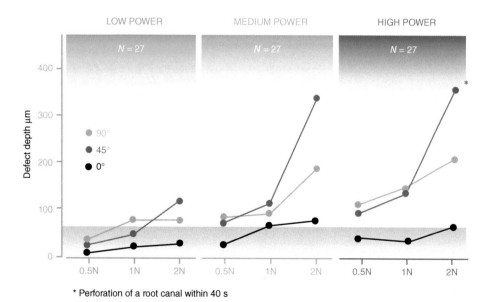

* Perforation of a root canal within 40 s

Figure 6.20 Effect of all combinations of lateral force and tip angulation at different power settings on defect depth after 40 seconds of instrumentation using a piezoelectric scaler. The shaded area indicates combinations of working parameters resulting in a clinically acceptable defect depth of less than 50 μm (*Source*: Flemmig et al., 1998a. Adapted with permission of John Wiley & Sons)

ULTRASONIC INSTRUMENTATION TECHNIQUE

a low–medium power setting and 0° angulation. And as previously noted, these conclusions were made prior to the publication of studies demonstrating the influence of tip shape on root surface damage (Jepsen et al., 2004; Lea et al., 2009b). Given what is now known regarding the influence of tip shape on root surface alteration, it is highly likely that the differences between piezoelectric and magnetostrictive units observed by Flemmig et al. in regard to lateral pressure and root surface alteration may, too, be due to the differences in tip shape rather than generator type, with the broad/flat tip used on the piezoelectric unit (Figure 6.16a) being more aggressive, particularly when applied with increasing lateral force, than the cylindrical tip used with the magnetostrictive unit (Figure 6.16b).

Assuming 0–15° tip angulation and a power setting appropriate for the task at hand, the degree of lateral force which keeps root surface damage to a minimum while maximizing the efficiency of deposit removal will vary between 0.5 and 2 N, depending on type of deposit to be removed:

- Minimal lateral force (0.5 N) should be applied during the scaling of calculus with wide diameter tips to minimize damage to the root surface.

- When performing debridement of biofilm with a slim diameter tip, a slightly greater degree of lateral force (1 to 2 N) should be applied to optimize the occurrence of cavitation at the active area of the tip.

Clinically, such an objective measurement of lateral force, in Newtons, cannot be made, requiring the clinician to rely on an arbitrary indication of force instead. An arbitrary indication of lateral force, such as "light," is subjective and thus will vary among clinicians. The mean amount of lateral force typically applied by practicing clinicians during ultrasonic instrumentation has been found to range between 0.2 and 1.34 N, with dental hygienists applying a mean force of 0.77 (±0.28) N, and dentists applying a mean force of 1.00 (±0.25) N (Ruppert et al., 2002).

To facilitate some measure of consistency among clinicians, the minimal degree of lateral force (0.5 N) might be described as one that "just keeps the tip in contact with the tooth surface," similar to, if not slightly less than, the force applied to explore a tooth surface.

To estimate the maximum 1–2 N of lateral force, by comparison, "pressure slightly greater than that used for an exploratory stroke" or "significantly less than (or one-fifth) the force applied to a hand scaler" may resonate.

Working stroke

The term *working stroke* is used to designate the stroke activated by the clinician, as opposed to the stroke inherent to the oscillating tip.

In order to optimize the effectiveness of the ultrasonic mechanisms of action, the working stroke needs to navigate the tip through the treatment site with a deliberate and methodical intent to make contact with every square millimeter of the involved tooth surfaces. Insufficient stroking, particularly nonoverlapping strokes, has been implicated as the principal cause of incomplete deposit removal in sites where instrumentation is not impeded by anatomic obstacles (Breininger et al., 1987) (Box 6.2).

Box 6.2: Key point

Insufficient stroking, particularly nonoverlapping strokes, is the principal cause of incomplete deposit removal in sites where instrumentation is not impeded by anatomic obstacles!

Proper ultrasonic stroking technique generates a working stroke which may be likened to an "*erasing*" motion, in that the stroking is bi-directional, equally distributed, short, overlapping, and constant. These elements are detailed and illustrated in Box 6.3.

Box 6.3: Characteristics of the ultrasonic working stroke

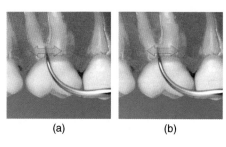

(a)   (b)

Figure 6.21 The ultrasonic working stroke is (a) bi-directional, such as forward and backward, and distributed equally in both directions; (b) avoid making one direction more prominent, or longer, than the other. (Length of stroke, as indicated by arrow, is exaggerated for visual ease)

Bi-directional: Because of the multiple mechanisms of action produced by the oscillating tip, deposit disruption and removal occurs regardless of the direction of the working stroke. Accordingly, ultrasonic working strokes are bi-directional, such as forward and backward (Figure 6.21a), or upward and downward, as the backward or downward strokes are as effective at disrupting/removing the deposits as the forward or upward strokes. This is in contrast to the working stroke of a manual instrument, where the cutting edge is stroked in one direction only, apico-coronally, to break the deposit from the tooth.

Equally distributed: The distance the tip is moved in each direction of the bi-directional stroke should be equal; the forward or upward motion should not be longer than the backward or downward motion (Figure 6.21b).

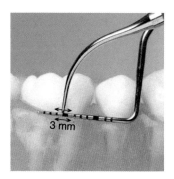

Figure 6.22 The length of the bi-directional working stroke should not exceed 2–3 mm in total

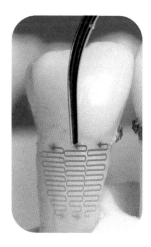

Figure 6.23 Overlapping pattern of the working stroke used to advance the tip in/out of the pocket and across the involved surface

Short: To ensure that the oscillating tip adequately contacts every square millimeter of the involved tooth surface, the bi-directional working stroke should not exceed 2–3 mm in total length (0.5–1.5 mm in each direction), with even shorter strokes necessary in narrow areas or pockets (Figure 6.22).

Overlapping: The working strokes should overlap as the tip is advanced in and out of the pocket, as well as across the surface of the tooth being treated (Figure 6.23).

Constant: The oscillating tip needs to stay in constant motion to prevent frictional heating that may be uncomfortable for the patient and damaging to the tooth; never allow the tip to idle on any one spot. Control of a tip in motion is more important than the speed of the motion. For students just beginning to develop instrumentation skills, stroking can be performed slowly, but continually; speed of stroking will increase as skill level progresses.

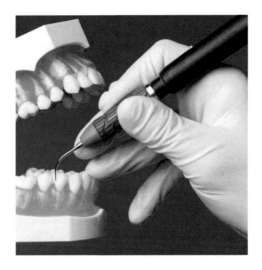

Figure 6.24 Flex the thumb, index, and middle fingers to digitally activate the ultrasonic working stroke

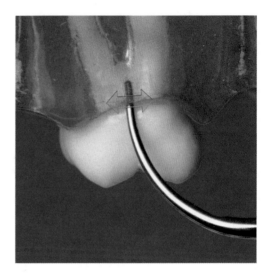

Figure 6.25 Horizontal working stroke

Table 6.3 Ultrasonic instrumentation working strokes

Stroke direction	Indication for use
Horizontal	Vertical adaptation on buccal/facial and lingual crown and root surfaces
Oblique	Vertical adaptation on interproximal root surfaces; Oblique adaptation on any surface
Vertical	Horizontal adaptation on interproximal crown surfaces; Vertical adaptation in narrow pocket
Tapping	Tenacious or heavy supragingival calculus

The motion of the working stroke is activated digitally by flexing the thumb, index, and middle fingers, as is done during periodontal probing and exploring (Figure 6.24). *Digital activation* is indicated and acceptable when the physical strength of the clinician is not required for deposit removal (Nield-Gehrig, 2008), whereas wrist activation is indicated to remove deposits with manual instruments.

The pattern, or direction, of the working strokes implemented by the clinician will vary depending upon the tooth surface being treated and the method of adaptation. Indications for using the various stroke directions are summarized in Table 6.3.

A. Horizontal stroke

With the oscillating tip adapted vertically to the buccal/facial and lingual tooth surfaces, the active area of the tip is methodically stroked across the treatment site in a *horizontal* (left–right) direction, as illustrated in Figure 6.25.

B. Oblique stroke

When the oscillating tip is adapted vertically on an interproximal root surface, a

ULTRASONIC INSTRUMENTATION TECHNIQUE

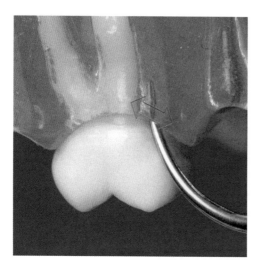

Figure 6.26 Oblique working stroke

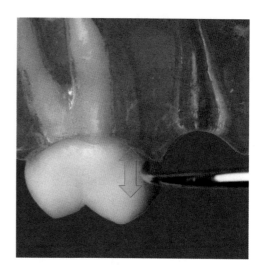

Figure 6.27 Vertical working stroke

methodical *oblique* (diagonal) stroke is used to advance the active area across the proximal surface of the root (Figure 6.26). An oblique stroke is also indicated if the tip is adapted to any tooth surface in an oblique orientation, as may be the case when limited access makes attaining true vertical adaptation difficult.

C. Vertical stroke

A *vertical* (up–down) stroke is used primarily to scale/debride the proximal surface of a crown when the back or face of the active area is adapted in a horizontal orientation (Figure 6.27). Vertical strokes may also be used with a tip in vertical adaptation to debride very narrow pockets.

D. Tapping stroke

A *tapping* stroke is only indicated to be used on tenacious, supragingival calculus. With a tapping stroke, the point of the oscillating tip is gently "tapped" against the calculus, using the high energy inherent to the point to break apart the tenacious calculus (Figure 6.28). As explained in Chapter 4, Tip Design and Selection, the point of the ultrasonic tip should never be directed against the root surface, as severe root damage is likely to result.

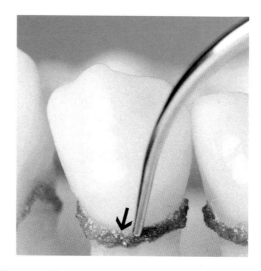

Figure 6.28 Tapping stroke (supragingival use only)

Insertion and advancement

Because ultrasonic mechanisms of action disrupt and obliterate deposits as the tip engages the deposit (Chapter 3), stroking begins at the gingival margin of the pocket for subgingival instrumentation (Figure 6.29a), or at an outermost edge of a supragingival deposit (Figure 6.29b). This is in contrast to the manual instrumentation technique, which requires the

ULTRASONIC INSTRUMENTATION TECHNIQUE

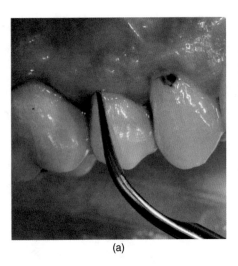 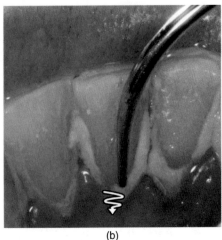

(a)   (b)

Figure 6.29 Insertion: stroking begins at (a) the gingival margin for subgingival instrumentation or (b) any edge of a supragingival deposit

cutting edge to be inserted below the calculus in order to break the bond between the calculus and tooth when the working stroke is activated.

With insertion beginning at the gingival margin, the tip must be advanced subgingivally in a manner that increases the predictability of the active area of the tip (terminal 3–4 mm) contacting all segments of the involved tooth surface. In pockets deeper than the length of the active area (>4 mm), this is accomplished by *channeling*. With channeling, the tip is advanced to the base of the pocket using a series of short, overlapping horizontal or oblique strokes, as previously indicated. Upon reaching the base of the pocket, the tip is then retreated out of the pocket by methodically stroking back toward the gingival margin, following the same path used for insertion before advancing proximally to debride the next *channel* (Figure 6.30).

This channel-like approach avoids a technique error easily made, which results in incomplete subgingival instrumentation (Figure 6.31). Because the active area is limited to the terminal 3–4 mm of the tip, if the tip is inserted to the base of the deep pocket and advanced proximally from that depth, the active tip area fails to contact, and subsequently debride, the root surface area coronal to the active area of the tip (shown shaded in Figure 6.31).

Grasp

While a firm, modified pen grasp of a bladed instrument is required for stabilization and control during the wrist-activated motion of manual instrumentation, a *light, pen grasp* of the ultrasonic handpiece facilitates digital activation and is essential to minimize the amount of lateral pressure applied, maximize the clinician's tactile sensitivity, and be ergonomically favorable for the clinician. To determine the correct position of grasp on the ultrasonic handpiece, the clinician should first balance the handpiece between the thumb and index finger (Figure 6.32a). From this point of balance, the clinician then wraps the thumb, index, and middle fingers down into a standard pen grasp (Figure 6.32b,c) .

With magnetostrictive instruments, the pen grasp should spread between the grip of the insert and the handpiece (Figure 6.32b). An error in grasp occurs when the clinician grasps only the magnetostrictive insert grip with all three fingers (Figure 6.33a) or the piezoelectric handpiece in very close proximity to the tip (Figure 6.33b). A grasp this close to the tip makes it difficult for the clinician to stabilize the handpiece in a manner that facilitates proper ultrasonic adaptation and stroking techniques.

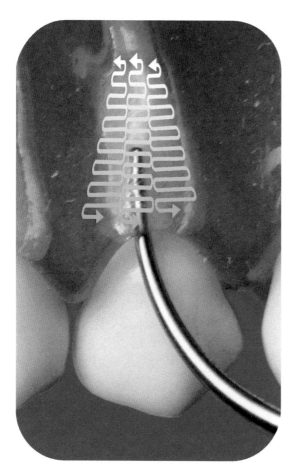

Figure 6.30 *Channeling.* Advancing the tip over the treatment surface in channels optimizes contact of the tip with all segments of the involved surface

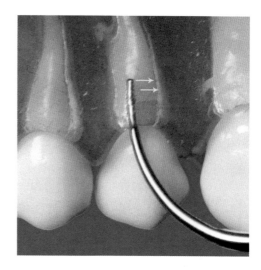

Figure 6.31 If the tip is advanced proximally from the base of the pocket, the active area of the tip fails to contact the area of root surface shaded in this image, resulting in incomplete deposit removal

Tactile sensitivity is the ability to distinguish tooth irregularities through the sense of touch. Tactile sensitivity develops with experience and is influenced by instrument design and clinician grasp, with a relaxed grasp and light lateral pressure required for optimal proprioception. In comparing the benefits and limitations of ultrasonic and hand instrumentation, it is commonly accepted (and perhaps assumed) that clinicians experience less tactile sensitivity with the use of ultrasonic instruments than with hand instruments. Although available evidence specific to this topic is minimal, it does not support this viewpoint. Tactile sensitivity significantly increased with ultrasonic scaling and

decreased with hand-activated scaling over a 45-minute period of use by first year dental hygiene students when objectively measured by a vibratory sensory analyzer (VSA) (Ryan et al., 2005). Subjectively, experienced clinicians have reported an equal or greater ability to feel attachment levels and root irregularities with slim diameter ultrasonic tips than with hand instruments (Dragoo, 1992).

The cord of the handpiece tends to weigh the end of the handpiece down, making the handpiece feel heavy to the clinician. Figures 6.34a and 6.34b illustrate a few tactics to managing the cord in order to reduce the pull on the handpiece or keep it from interfering with the instrumentation procedure.

Features on newer ultrasonic scaling units designed to minimize cord pull and cord interference include swiveling connections between the handpiece and cord, cords lighter in weight, and/or cords with greater flexibility.

Fulcrum

During ultrasonic instrumentation, a fulcrum is needed to stabilize the clinician's grasp on the handpiece, not to provide leverage for a working

ULTRASONIC INSTRUMENTATION
TECHNIQUE

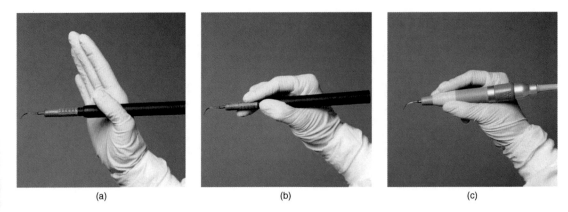

(a) (b) (c)

Figure 6.32 To determine the correct position of the standard pen grasp, (a) the ultrasonic handpiece is first balanced between the thumb and index finger. At the point of balance, the thumb, index, and middle fingers are laid down into a standard pen grasp of the (b) magnetostrictive or (c) piezoelectric handpiece

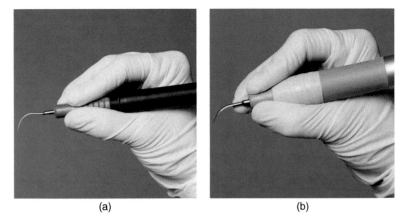

(a) (b)

Figure 6.33 An error in grasp occurs if all fingers rest (a) on the grip of a magnetostrictive insert or (b) in close proximity to the piezoelectric tip

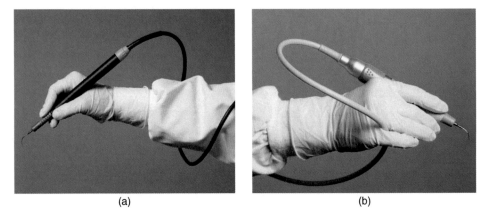

(a) (b)

Figure 6.34 Tactics to manage the handpiece cord or reduce cord pull include (a) loosely wrapping the cord around the forearm or (b) grasping a slack of cord between the ring and little fingers

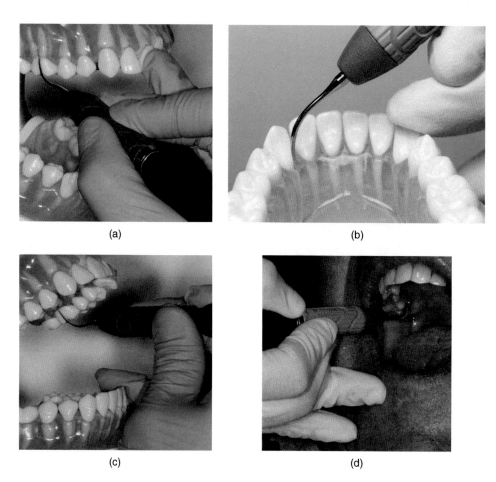

(a)

(b)

(c)

(d)

Figure 6.35 Fulcrums which provide stabilization at a distance from the treatment site: (a) the *split fulcrum* is established in the same quadrant as the treatment site, but requires no contact between the middle and ring fingers; (b) the *cross-arch fulcrum* is similar to the split fulcrum, established in the same arch as the treatment site but in the other quadrant; (c) the *opposite-arch fulcrum* is established on the arch opposite of the treatment site; (d) the *extraoral fulcrum* is established on facial surfaces, such as the cheek or border of the mandible

stroke, as is required with hand instrumentation. As only stabilization, not leverage, is needed, the clinician has greater flexibility in establishing fulcrum positions than with hand instrumentation. The goal is to find a point of stabilization that enables the clinician to maintain appropriate adaptation of the tip as it is advanced across all surfaces of the treatment area. This stabilization point is typically more distant from the treatment site than fulcrums used during manual instrumentation. As such, the use of alternative fulcrums, such as *split* (Figure 6.35a) or *cross arch* (Figure 6.35b) fulcrums on the same arch

as the treatment site, are recommended over a standard intraoral rest, with *opposite arch* (Figure 6.35c), and *extraoral* (Figure 6.35d) fulcrums being acceptable options.

AEROSOL MANAGEMENT

It was explained in Section 3.3 that all ultrasonic instruments are operated with a continuous supply of water flowing over the oscillating tip to act as a coolant and reduce frictional heat. The interaction between the high-frequency tip vibrations

ULTRASONIC INSTRUMENTATION TECHNIQUE

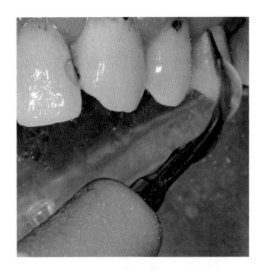

Figure 6.36 Aerosol generated by an ultrasonic tip oscillating at a higher power for scaling of calculus

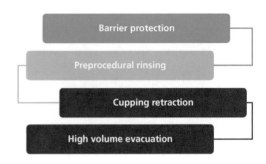

Figure 6.37 Protective steps, or layers, to minimize cross-contamination by the aerosol generated during ultrasonic instrumentation

and the flowing water produces an aerosol, or fine mist, with the degree of aerosolization influenced by power setting and water flow rate.

Specific to infection control, *aerosols* are defined as airborne suspensions of solid or liquid particles smaller than 50 μm, with suspensions of particles larger than 50 μm being described as *splatter* (Harrel et al., 1998; Rivera-Hidalgo et al., 1999).

Ultrasonic and sonic instruments generate both aerosols and splatter regardless of volume of coolant water used (Gross et al., 1992), with blood and bacteria from the treatment site contaminating the suspensions (Holbrook et al., 1978; Fine et al., 1992; Gross et al., 1992; Bentley et al., 1994; Grenier 1995; Barnes et al., 1998), creating a vehicle for the transmission of blood-borne pathogens (Figure 6.36). Therefore, methods to manage the aerosol and splatter in order to minimize cross-contamination are a fundamental component of ultrasonic instrumentation technique.

Minimizing cross-contamination from the aerosol requires what Harrel and Molinari (2004) refer to as a *layering of protective procedures*, with risk of aerosol contamination being further reduced with every step,

or layer, taken until the risk is minimal. The protective steps recommended to minimize cross-contamination by the aerosol generated during ultrasonic instrumentation are summarized in Figure 6.37.

Barrier protection

As the use of personal barrier protection (protective eyewear for both the clinician and patient, masks, gloves, and cover gowns) is mandated during all dental procedures in the United States by the 1991 Occupational Safety and Health Administration's (OSHA) Standard on Occupational Exposure to Bloodborne Pathogens, the specifics of such basic infection control measures will not be addressed in this textbook. Relatedly, the United States Centers for Disease Control and Prevention (CDC) Guidelines for Infection Control in Dental Health-Care Settings (Kohn et al., 2003) recommend that surface barrier protection be used to prevent contamination of clinical contact surfaces, which cannot be adequately cleaned by sterilization or disinfection.

Preprocedural rinsing

Rinsing with an essential oil antiseptic mouthwash for 30 seconds prior to ultrasonic instrumentation has been shown to reduce the level of recoverable viable bacteria in the aerosol generated by 94% (Fine et al., 1992).

Likewise, a preprocedural rinse using 0.12% chlorhexidine gluconate significantly reduced the bacterial count in the saliva (Veksler et al., 1991) and in the aerosol generated during ultrasonic instrumentation (Klyn et al., 2001).

While the preprocedural rinse may effectively reduce contamination of the aerosol by the free-floating microorganisms in the saliva and oral cavity, it will not eliminate contamination of the aerosol by the blood and bacteria that arise during instrumentation of the subgingival treatment site (Harrel and Molinari, 2004). To reduce the contamination arising from the operative site, as much of the aerosol as possible should be physically removed before it escapes the immediate treatment site (Harrel and Molinari, 2004).

Cupping retraction

In an effort to keep the aerosol somewhat contained in the oral cavity until it can be removed, the lips and cheeks in the treatment area should be retracted using a *cupping* technique. Retracting the patient's lip or cheek by pulling it out, then up or down (lips) or forward (cheek), forms a cup that keeps the aerosol from escaping by deflecting it back into the oral cavity. See Figure 6.38.

High-volume evacuation

High-volume evacuation (HVE) has been shown to reduce the aerosol produced during ultrasonic instrumentation by more than 90% (Harrel et al., 1996; Klyn et al., 2001; Jacks, 2002). HVE systems remove a large volume of air within a short period (up to 100 cubic feet of air per minute) and typically have a large bore (≥8 mm) (Harrel and Molinari, 2004). A saliva ejector, which has a small bore, is ineffective in removing aerosols and should only be used to remove water accumulation from the oral cavity (Jacks, 2002).

When suctioning with HVE, the inlet of the HVE attachment needs to be held close enough to the source of aerosols to evacuate those aerosols (10–20 mm), while avoiding contact of the HVE attachment with the ultrasonic instrument and the patient's intra-oral tissues (Mamoun, 2011). For the clinician working alone, without a dental assistant, this can be a difficult and cumbersome task to accomplish, especially if using the traditionally long and straight HVE attachments. Jacks (2002) found an extra-oral hands-free HVE attachment positioned within one inch of the commissure of the patient's lip to be just as effective as the traditional intra-orally

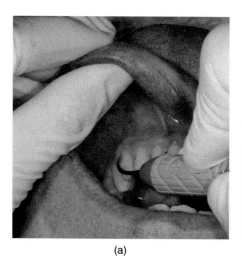
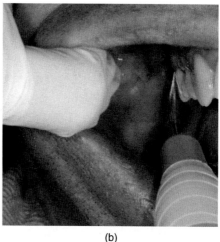

(a)   (b)

Figure 6.38 Retraction of (a) the lower lip (from clinician's viewpoint) and (b) the cheek to form a "cup," which helps contain the aerosol within the oral cavity where it can be evacuated

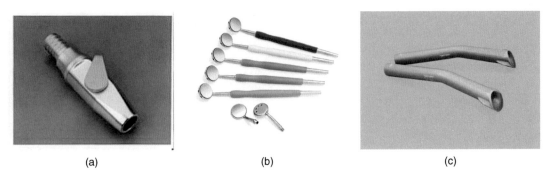

(a)   (b)   (c)

Figure 6.39 (a) BullFrog® aluminum lightweight HVE handpiece – short; (b) mirror/suction device for HVE; (c) Pelotte® angled evacuation tips (Images courtesy of Hager Worldwide)

positioned HVE attachment in removing the aerosol generated during ultrasonic debridement. Unfortunately, such a hands free device is not commercially available at the time of this writing. Newer HVE devices currently available offer modifications, such as lighter weight, shorter length, angled configuration, and/or mirrored surfaces, which ease use of the HVE by the sole practitioner. Figure 6.39 illustrates several of these products.

Even with proper utilization of the HVE, some aerosol will escape into the operatory air (Jacks, 2002; Timmerman et al., 2004). To reduce the aerosols that have escaped into the operatory air, the HVE suction should remain on continuously during the entire debridement procedure, even during momentary stops in instrumentation, and should be kept on for a few minutes after the procedure is completed (Mamoun, 2011).

Other options available to the clinician working alone include an HVE aerosol reduction device (ARD) that attaches directly to the ultrasonic handpiece (Figure 6.40) or a multifunctional isolation device, which provides illumination and retraction in addition to high volume aspiration (Figure 6.41).

Attaching the HVE ARD directly to the ultrasonic handpiece has been demonstrated to significantly reduce aerosol contamination during ultrasonic scaling (Harrel et al., 1996; Klyn et al.,

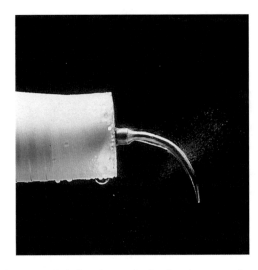

Figure 6.40 Safety Suction®, Quality Aspirators (Image courtesy of Stephen K. Harrel, DDS)

2001), and more so than the use of a preoperative chlorhexidine rinse alone (Klyn et al., 2001). However, combining the ARD with the preoperative chlorhexidine rinse was no more effective than the use of the ARD alone (Klyn et al., 2001).

STAGED APPROACH TO ULTRASONIC INSTRUMENTATION

By this point, it has been established that the objectives of periodontal debridement therapy

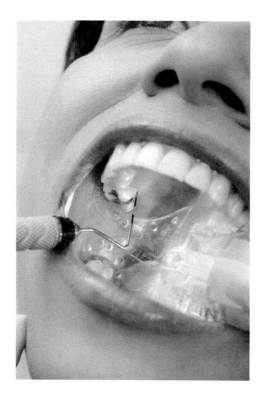

Figure 6.41 Isolite™ i2 Dryfield Illuminator System (Image courtesy of Isolite Systems)

the removal of biofilm (Flemmig et al., 1998a,b), instrumentation must be implemented in two stages (Box 6.4), as initially proposed by Kieser (Chapter 1).

Box 6.4: Stages of Instrumentation

Scaling: Instrumentation aimed at reducing moderate–heavy and/or tenacious calculus deposits to a lesser degree

Debridement: Instrumentation aimed at the definitive removal of biofilm, and remaining calculus, without intentional cementum removal

---

Scaling stage

When moderate–heavy and/or tenacious calculus deposits predominate the treatment site, such as in initial periodontal therapy (Figure 6.42), instrumentation begins with the scaling stage.

The term *scaling* refers to the process of removing calculus (O'Leary, 1986). The objective of

are to create an environment conducive to healing by thorough disruption of all deposits, without over-instrumentation of the root surface. It has also been established that accomplishing these objectives by means of ultrasonic instrumentation is contingent upon a number of synergistic working parameters, including operational (power setting, water flow rate) and technique (tip design, angulation, adaptation, and lateral pressure) variables.

Implementing effective ultrasonic instrumentation requires the clinician to comprehend the synergistic relationship of these working parameters and adjust the variables as appropriate for the task at hand; the task at hand being the type of deposit to be removed. As the effective and efficient removal of calculus deposits requires different working parameters than does

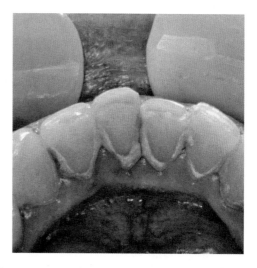

Figure 6.42 Moderate–heavy calculus deposits are removed or reduced during the scaling stage of periodontal therapy

ULTRASONIC INSTRUMENTATION TECHNIQUE

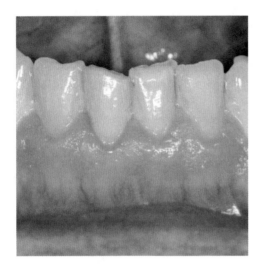

Figure 6.43 The presence of biofilm and minimal calculus deposits indicate the need for debridement instrumentation

Debridement stage

When biofilm and/or minimal calculus predominate the treatment site (Figure 6.43), as in the case of supportive periodontal therapy (SPT), prophylaxis, and upon completion of the scaling stage of initial therapy, debridement instrumentation is indicated.

The term *debridement* refers to the process of removing light calculus, biofilm, and endotoxin in a conservative manner (Smart et al., 1990). The objective of debridement instrumentation is to definitively remove these deposits while being careful to avoid over-instrumentation of the root surface, that is, in a conservative manner. This requires working parameters that are low enough to prevent root damage but high enough to efficiently remove the biofilm and light calculus (Flemmig et al., 1998a,b). These constraints are met by using a slim or ultraslim cylindrically shaped tip within the range of medium-low to medium power and with slightly more lateral force applied than when performing ultrasonic scaling of calculus.

the scaling stage is to reduce substantial calculus deposits to a lesser degree. The scaling stage may also be described as the gross, meaning unrefined, removal of calculus.

To accomplish scaling of calculus in the most efficient manner, the use of a standard diameter tip, cylindrical or rectangular in shape, within the range of medium to medium–high power and adapted with the slightest degree of lateral force is indicated.

Guidelines for the working parameters of each stage of ultrasonic instrumentation are summarized in Table 6.4. Practical application of these guidelines is demonstrated in the case studies presented in Chapter 8.

Table 6.4 Working parameters for the stages of ultrasonic instrumentation

Working parameter	Scaling stage	Debridement stage
Tip diameter	Standard	Slim or ultraslim
Tip shape/alignment	Cylindrical or rectangular; straight	Cylindrical; straight or curved (depending on site anatomy)
Power setting	Medium to med-high	Med-low to medium
Lateral pressure	≤ Exploratory (0.5 N)	> Exploratory (1–2 N) < Manual Scaling
Angulation	0–15°	0–15°

REFERENCES

Barnes JB, Harrel SK, Rivera-Hidalgo F. Blood contamination of the aerosols produced by in vivo use of ultrasonic scalers. *J Periodontol* 1998; 69: 434–48.

Bentley CD, Burkhart NW, Crawford JJ. Evaluating spatter and aerosol contamination during dental procedures. *J Am Dent Assoc* 1994; 125: 579–84.

Breininger DR, O'Leary TJ, Blumenshine RVH. Comparative effectiveness of ultrasonic and hand scaling for the removal of subgingival plaque and calculus. *J Periodontol* 1987; 58: 9–18.

Busslinger A, Lampe K, Buechat M, Lehmann B. A comparative in vitro study of a magnetostrictive and a piezoelectric ultrasonic scaling instrument. *J Clin Periodontol* 2001; 28:642–9.

Dragoo MR. A clinical evaluation of hand and ultrasonic instruments on subgingival debridement. Part 1. With unmodified and modified ultrasonic inserts. *Int J Periodontics Restorative Dent* 1992; 12: 310–23.

Felver B, King DC, Lea SC, Price GJ, Walmsley AD. Cavitation occurrence around ultrasonic dental scalers. *Ultrason Sonochem* 2009; 16: 692–7.

Fine DH, Mendieta C, Barnett ML, Furgang D, Meyers R, Olshan A, Vincent J. Efficacy of preprocedural rinsing with an antiseptic in reducing viable bacteria in dental aerosols. *J Periodontol* 1992; 63: 821–4.

Flemmig TF, Petersilka GJ, Mehl A, Rudiger S, Hickel R, Klaiber B. Working parameters of a sonic scaler influencing root substance removal in vitro. *Clin Oral Invest* 1997; 1:55–60.

Flemmig TF, Petersilka GJ, Mehl A, Hickel R, Klaiber B. The effect of working parameters on root substance removal using a piezoelectric ultrasonic scaler in vitro. *J Clin Periodontol* 1998a; 25: 158–63.

Flemmig TF, Petersilka GJ, Mehl A, Hickel R, Klaiber B. Working parameters of a magnetostrictive ultrasonic scaler influencing root substance removal in vitro. *J Periodontol* 1998b; 69: 547–53. 165–68.

Grenier D. Quantitative analysis of bacterial aerosols in two different clinic environments. *Appl Environ Microbiol* 1995; 61: 3165–8.

Gross KB, Overman PR, Cobb C, Brockman S. Aerosol generation by two ultrasonic scalers and one sonic scaler: a comparative study. *J Dent Hyg* 1992; 66: 314–8.

Harrel SK, Barnes JB, Rivera-Hidalgo F. Reduction of aerosols produced by ultrasonic scalers. *J Periodontol* 1996; 67: 28–32.

Harrel SK, Barnes JB, Rivera-Hidalgo F. Aerosol and splatter contamination from the operative site during ultrasonic scaling. *J Am Dent Assoc* 1998; 129: 1241–9.

Holbrook WP, Muir KF, MacPhee IT, Ross PW. Bacteriological investigation of the aerosol from ultrasonic scalers. *Br Dent J* 1978; 144: 245–7.

Jacks ME. A laboratory comparison of evacuation devices on aerosol reduction. *J Dent Hyg* 2002; 76: 202–6.

Jacobson L, Blomlof J, Lindskog S. Root surface texture after different scaling modalities. *Scand J Dent Res* 1994; 102: 156–60.

Jepsen S, Ayna M, Hedderich J, Eberhard J. Significant influence of scaler tip design on root substance loss resulting from ultrasonic scaling: a laserprofilometric in vitro study. *J Clin Periodontol* 2004; 31: 1003–6.

Kawashima H, Sato S, Kishida M, Ito K. A comparison of root surface instrumentation using two piezoelectric ultrasonic scalers and a hand scaler in vivo. *J Periodontal Res* 2007; 42: 90–5.

Khambay BS, Walmsley AD. Acoustic microstreaming detection and measurement around ultrasonic scalers. *J Periodontol* 1999; 70: 626–31.

Klyn S, Cummings D, Richardson B, Davis R. Reduction of bacteria-containing spray produced during ultrasonic scaling. *Gen Dent* 2001; 49: 648–52.

Kohn WG, Harte JA, Malvitz DM, Collins AS, Cleveland JL, Eklund KJ. Guidelines for infection control in dental health care settings – 2003. *J Am Dent Assoc* 2004; 135: 33–47.

Lea SC, Landini G, Walmsley AD. Ultrasonic scaler tip performance under various load conditions. *J Clin Periodontol* 2003; 30: 876–81.

Lea SC, Felver B, Landini G, Walmsley AD. Three-dimensional analyses of ultrasonic scaler oscillations. *J Clin Periodontol* 2009a; 36: 44–50.

Lea SC, Felver B, Landini G, Walmsley AD. Ultrasonic scaler oscillations and tooth-surface defects. *J Dent Res* 2009b; 88: 229–34.

Lea SC, Walmsley AD. Mechano-physical and biophysical properties of power-driven scalers: driving the future of powered instrument design and evaluation. *Periodontol 2000* 2009; 51: 63–78.

Mamoun JS. Clinical techniques of performing suctioning tasks and of positioning the HVE attachment and inlet when assisting a dentist. A guide for dental assistants Part 1. *Dent Assist* 2011; 80: 38–40, 42–4, 46.

Nield-Gehrig, JS. (2008) *Fundamentals of periodontal instrumentation and advanced root instrumentation.* Lippincott Williams & Wilkins, Baltimore.

O'Leary TJ. The impact of research on scaling and root planing. *J Periodontol* 1986; 57: 69–75.

Ritz, L, Hefti AF, Rateitschak KH. An in vitro investigation on the loss of root substance in scaling with various instruments. *J Clin Periodontol* 1991; 18: 643–47.

Rivera-Hidalgo F, Barnes JB, Harrel SK. Aerosol and splatter reduction by focused spray and standard ultrasonic inserts. *J Periodontol* 1999; 70: 473–7.

Ruppert M, Cadosch J, Guindy J, Case D, Zappa U. In vivo ultrasonic debridement force in bicuspids: a pilot study. *J Periodontol* 2002; 73: 418–22.

Ryan DL, Darby M, Bauman D, Tolle SL, Naik D. Effects of ultrasonic scaling and hand-activated scaling on tactile sensitivity in dental hygiene students. *J Dent Hyg* 2005; 79: 9.

Schmidlin P, Beuchat M, Busslinger A, Lehmann B, Lutz F. Tooth substance loss resulting from mechanical, sonic and ultrasonic root instrumentation assessed by liquid scintillation. *J Clin Periodontol* 2001; 28: 1058–66.

Smart GJ, Wilson M, Davies EH, Kieser JB. The assessment of ultrasonic root surface debridement by determination of residual endotoxin levels. *J Clin Periodontal* 1990; 17: 174–8.

Timmerman M, Menso L, Steinfort J, van Winkelhoff AJ, van der Weijden GA. Atmospheric contamination during ultrasonic scaling; *J Clin Periodontol* 2004; 31: 458–62.

Trenter SC, Landini G, Walmsley AD. Effect of loading on the vibration characteristics of thin magnetostrictive ultrasonic scaler inserts. *J Periodontol* 2003; 74: 1308–15.

US Department of Labor, Occupational Safety and Health Administration. 29 CFR Part 1910.1030. Occupational exposure to bloodborne pathogens; needlesticks and other sharps injuries; final rule. *Federal Register* 2001; 66: 5317–25.

Veksler AE, Kayrouz GA, Newman MG. Reduction of salivary bacteria by pre-procedural rinses with chlorhexidine 0.12%. *J Periodontol* 1991; 62: 649–51.

Walmsley AD, Laird WRE, Williams AR. A model system to demonstrate the role of cavitational activity in ultrasonic scaling. *J Dent Res* 1984; 63: 1162–5.

Walmsley AD, Laird WRE, Williams AR. Dental plaque removal by cavitational activity during ultrasonic scaling. *J Clin Periodontol* 1988; 15: 539–43.

Walmsley AD, Lea SC, Felver B, King DC, Price GJ. Mapping cavitation activity around dental ultrasonic tips. *Clin Oral Invest* 2013; 17: 1227–34.

Zappa U, Cadosch J, Simona C, Graf H, Case D. In vivo scaling and root planing forces. *J Periodontol* 1991; 62: 335–40.

ULTRASONIC INSTRUMENTATION TECHNIQUE

Chapter 7
Ultrasonic instrumentation technique modules

CHAPTER OBJECTIVES

On completion of this chapter, the student will be able to:

1. Utilize instrumentation sequencing strategies that improve the efficiency of ultrasonic instrumentation.

2. Demonstrate appropriate implementation of each of the transitions in adaptation used to advance the ultrasonic tip through the treatment area.

3. Rationalize the preferential use of furcation-specific, ball-end tips for the debridement of furcational surfaces.

4. Execute proper ultrasonic instrumentation technique, using an appropriate tip design, in any area of the dentition.

In order to accomplish thorough debridement in the most efficient manner, the principles of ultrasonic instrumentation presented in Chapter 6 should be implemented in a systematic method or *sequence*. This chapter first addresses several strategies for instrumentation sequencing in general, followed by instructional technique and sequence modules specific to anterior and posterior sextants of the dentition, advanced furcation involvement, dental implants, and supragingival deposits.

STRATEGIES FOR INSTRUMENTATION SEQUENCING

Work by sextant

While it is common practice to treatment plan periodontal therapy by quadrant, ultrasonic instrumentation should be performed, in stages, by *sextant* (Figure 7.1), regardless of the extent of the treatment area (single quadrant, multiple quadrants, or full mouth).

As instrumentation of anterior and posterior teeth predictably require changes in regard to tip design and operator position, working by sextant reduces the frequency of changing these variables, resulting in a more efficient execution of instrumentation.

Likewise, when the presence of moderate–heavy calculus dictates two stages of instrumentation, as is frequently the case in initial periodontal therapy, completion of all scaling instrumentation, by sextant, throughout the designated treatment area before initiating any debridement instrumentation reduces the frequency of changing tip design per stage (scaling/debridement) and per location (anterior/posterior).

Ultrasonic Periodontal Debridement: Theory and Technique, First Edition. Marie D. George, Timothy G. Donley and Philip M. Preshaw.
© 2014 John Wiley & Sons, Inc. Published 2014 by John Wiley & Sons, Inc.

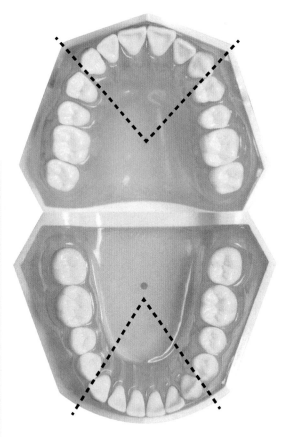

Figure 7.1 Division of the dentition into sextants; two anterior and four posterior sextants

Advance toward operator

Instrumentation in the designated treatment area should always advance toward the operator. This means in posterior sextants, for both left- and right-handed operators, instrumentation begins on the most posterior tooth and advances anteriorly, or toward the operator (Figure 7.2a). In anterior sextants, instrumentation begins on the tooth most distant from the operator, which differs according to handedness (left/right), and advances toward the operator (Figure 7.2b,c).

Points of adaptation

As with hand instrumentation, the *point of adaptation* (site on the tooth surface where

instrumentation will commence) is the midline of an anterior tooth (Figure 7.3a) and the distal line angle of the buccal and lingual surfaces of a posterior tooth (Figure 7.3b).

Unlike hand instrumentation, during which the bladed instrument is advanced through the treatment area by readapting the cutting edge at these points on each tooth, the ultrasonic tip is adapted at this point only on the first tooth in the designated treatment area to initiate an instrumentation sequence which advances by transitioning the tip to the adjacent surface, as described in the next section.

Box 7.1: "Proximal" versus "Interproximal": What's the difference?

The terms "proximal" and "interproximal" are used frequently throughout this chapter to distinguish different parts of the dentition. As these terms are often confused, it is important that they be defined prior to studying the remainder of this chapter.

Proximal: Nearest, next, immediately adjacent to; distal or mesial.

Proximal contact area: Proximal area on a tooth that touches an adjacent tooth; seen on the mesial or distal side.

Interproximal: between the proximal surfaces of adjoining teeth in the same arch.

Interproximal space: V-shaped spaces between the teeth formed by the proximal surfaces of adjoining teeth and their contact areas.

Advance by transitioning

Four fundamental *transitions* in adaptation are made to advance the oscillating tip through a designated treatment area in a sequence that optimizes the use of all surfaces of the tip, thus enabling thorough, efficient, and ergonomic instrumentation of all tooth surfaces.

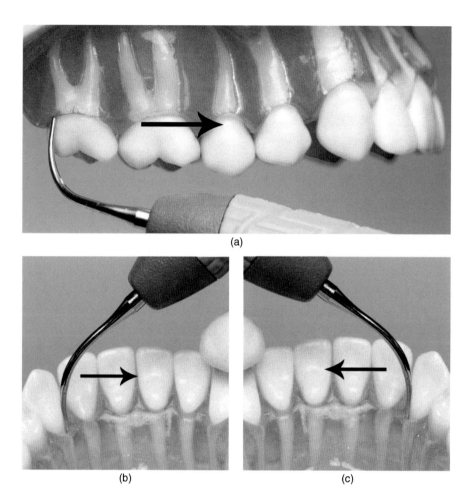

Figure 7.2 The sequence of instrumentation always advances towards the operator from (a) posterior to anterior or, in anterior sextants, from the tooth furthest from operator, which will differ for (b) right-handed versus (c) left-handed operators

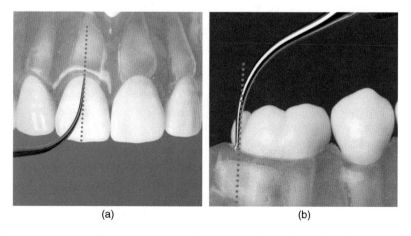

Figure 7.3 To initiate a sequence of instrumentation, the tip is adapted at (a) the midline of an anterior tooth and (b) the distal line angle of a posterior tooth

Figures 7.5–7.13 illustrate and describe each transition, with the blue arrow in each image indicating the direction of the working stroke used on each surface.

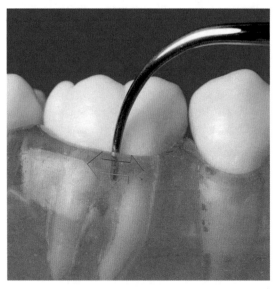

Starting from the primary position of vertical adaptation (as shown in Figure 7.3b), a lateral surface (or when applicable, the back) of the tip is advanced across buccal and lingual surfaces using horizontal strokes.

Figure 7.4 Lateral surface of tip vertically adapted to buccal surface. Arrow indicates horizontal stroke pattern

Transition to Proximal Root Surface: On reaching a line angle, vertical adaptation is maintained as the tip crosses the line angle to the proximal surface. On a mesial root surface, the back of the tip inherently adapts with this transition (Figure 7.5); on a distal root surface, the lateral surface of the tip remains adapted (Figure 7.6). The tip is then advanced across the proximal root surface using an oblique stroke pattern.

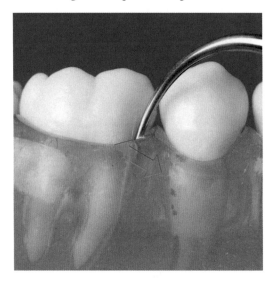

Figure 7.5 Back of tip vertically adapted to mesial surface. Arrow indicates oblique stroke pattern

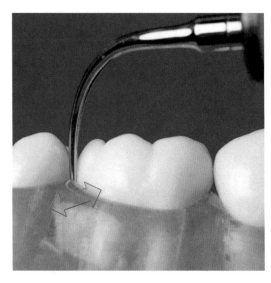

Figure 7.6 Lateral surface of tip vertically adapted to distal surface. Arrow indicates oblique stroke pattern

Box 7.2: Technique pointers

While the convex back of the tip is the ideal surface to adapt to concave root anatomy, it is not clinically possible on the distal aspect (Figure 7.7). Alternatively then, the lateral surface is used to debride the distal root surface (Figure 7.6).

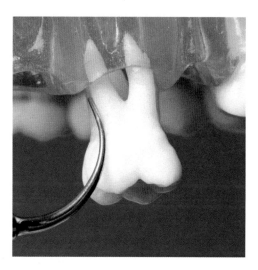

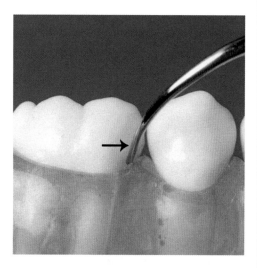

Figure 7.7 Although preferable, vertical adaptation of the convex back of the tip to the distal root anatomy is not clinically possible

Figure 7.8 Arrow indicates oblique adaptation of the lateral surface resulting from rotation of the tip at the line angle. Compare the position of the tip in this image to the preferable position illustrated in Figure 7.5

During subgingival instrumentation, DO NOT rotate the tip at the line angle, as is required during manual instrumentation. Rotating at the line angle *undesirably* transitions the tip from vertical adaptation of the preferred tip surface to oblique adaptation of a lateral surface (Figure 7.8), compromising access and contact of the tip to the proximal surface of the root.

Transition *to* Interproximal Space: As the interproximal space (or cervical embrasure) is entered, contact with the tooth is maintained while the tip is transitioned from vertical to horizontal adaptation by a slight rolling motion. On the distal aspect, the rolling motion adapts the face of the tip to the distal surface (Figure 7.9). On the mesial aspect, the back of the tip remains adapted to the mesial surface throughout this transition (Figure 7.10). *It is critical that this transition occurs in the interproximal space against enamel, rather than against root structure, to avoid severe root gouging by the point of the tip during the rolling motion.* Stroking of the back or face of the tip against the interproximal surface ensues in a vertical direction.

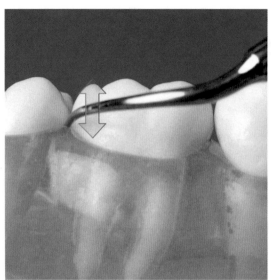

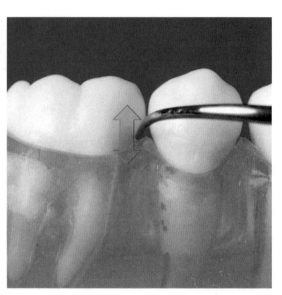

Figure 7.9 Horizontal adaptation of the face of the tip to the distal surface of the crown. Arrow indicates vertical stroke pattern

Figure 7.10 Horizontal adaptation of the back of the tip to mesial surface of the crown. Arrow indicates vertical stroke pattern

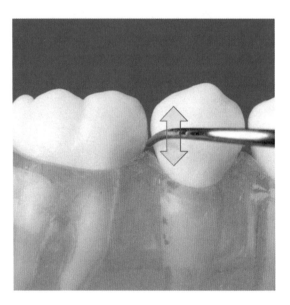

Figure 7.11 Instrumentation advances to the next tooth by horizontally adapting the face of the tip to the distal surface of the crown. Arrow indicates vertical stroke pattern

Transition to Next Tooth: Advancing from the mesial surface of one tooth to the next tooth in the treatment area is accomplished by maintaining horizontal orientation and bringing the face of the tip into adaptation with the distal surface of the adjacent tooth; stroke vertically against the distal surface.

Transition *from* **Interproximal Space:** Contact with the tooth is maintained as the tip is transitioned from horizontal to vertical adaptation by a slight rolling motion that adapts the lateral surface of the tip to the distal surface of the tooth (Figure 7.12). As with the transition to the interproximal space, *it is critical that this transition also occurs in the interproximal space against enamel to avoid severe root gouging by the point of the tip during the rolling motion.* The tip is then advanced subgingivally and stroked in an oblique direction over the distal root surface, toward the distal line angle (Figure 7.13).

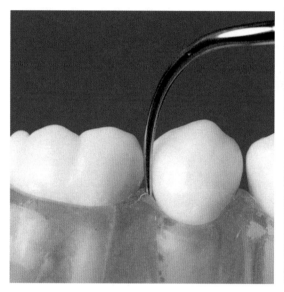
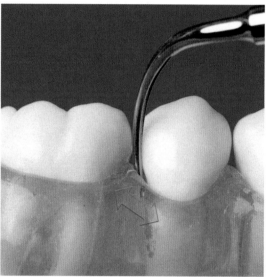

Figure 7.12 Vertical adaptation of the lateral surface of the tip to the distal surface of the tooth

Figure 7.13 After transitioning to vertical adaptation in the interproximal space, the tip is advanced subgingivally to the base of the pocket. Arrow indicates oblique stroke pattern

Utilization of these transitions in specific sextants of the dentition is described in the modules which follow.

ULTRASONIC INSTRUMENTATION TECHNIQUE MODULES

SEXTANT SPECIFIC INSTRUMENTATION MODULES

Step-by-step instructional modules for instrumentation of an anterior sextant (Module 1) and a posterior sextant (Module 2) are provided to exemplify the fundamental technique and sequence implemented throughout the dentition.

Although the tip design utilized will change according to the stage of instrumentation and anatomy of the treatment site (Chapter 4), the technique employed is common to all ultrasonic instruments. Thus, a variety of tips are shown throughout the modules to demonstrate universal application of the principles of ultrasonic technique and develop familiarity with an array of tip configurations.

Module 1
Anterior Sextant: Mandibular Anterior Lingual

Table 7.1 Operator position: mandibular anterior sextant (facial/lingual)

Operator	Preferred position	Alternative position
Right-handed		
	12:00	8:00
	Figure 7.14	Figure 7.15
Left-handed		
	12:00	4:00
	Figure 7.14	Figure 7.16

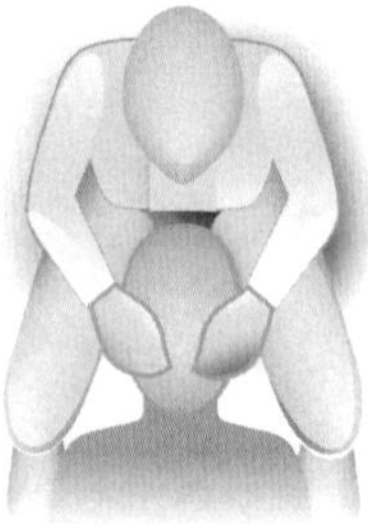

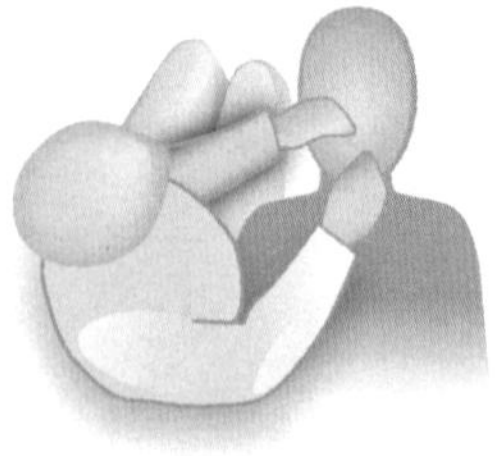

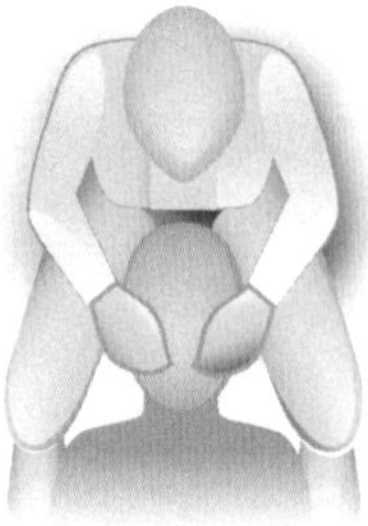

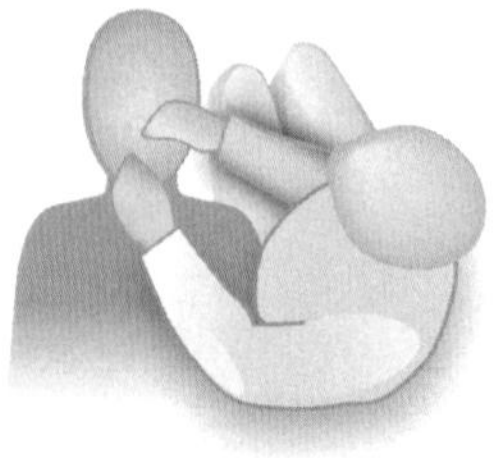

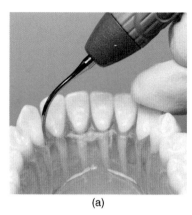 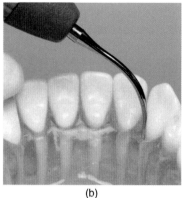

Begin at the tooth furthest away from operator: (a) #22 (FDI 33) for right-handed operators; (b) #27(FDI 43) for left-handed operators.

(a)   (b)

Figure 7.17

NOTE: Figures 7.18–7.27 illustrate the sequence for right-handed operators. Left-handed operators will follow the same sequence, but advancing through the sextant from the opposite direction.

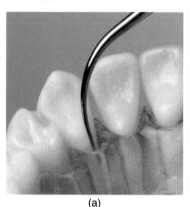 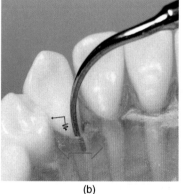

Vertically adapt lateral surface (or back) of active tip at the midline (i.e. point of adaptation). Implement horizontal strokes to advance tip subgingivally and distally toward DL line angle.

(a)   (b)

Figure 7.18 #22 (33) L: (a) ultra-thin straight tip (b) slim right curved tip; blue arrow indicates direction of the working stroke, black arrows indicate the path of tip advancement from this point

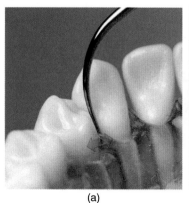 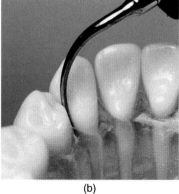

As tip crosses DL line angle, **transition to distal root surface** by maintaining vertical adaptation of lateral surface to distal aspect of tooth. Advance subgingivally and facially using horizontal or slightly oblique strokes until hindered by contact point.

(a)   (b)

Figure 7.19 #22 (33) D: (a) ultra-thin straight tip; (b) slim right curved tip

MODULE 1
ANTERIOR SEXTANT: MANDIBULAR
ANTERIOR LINGUAL

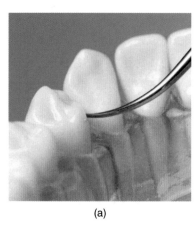
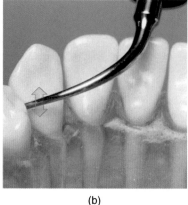

(a)   (b)

Transition *to* distal interprox-imal space by horizontally adapting face of tip to distal surface of #22 (FDI 33); stroke vertically.

Figure 7.20 #22 (33) D IP: (a) ultra-thin straight tip; (b) slim right curved tip

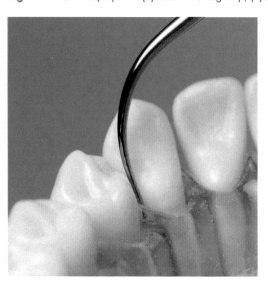

Transition *from* distal interproximal space by returning to vertical adaptation of the lateral surface; stroke to retreat tip to DL line angle.

Figure 7.21 #22 (33) D: ultra-thin straight tip

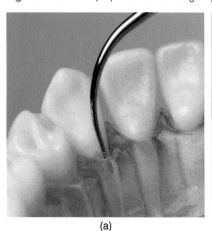
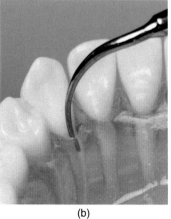

(a)   (b)

Cross DL line angle and proceed with horizontal strokes to advance tip subgingivally and mesially across lingual surface, toward ML line angle.

Figure 7.22 # 22 (33) L: (a) ultra-thin straight tip; (b) slim right curved tip

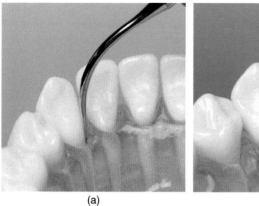
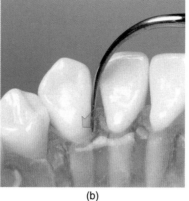

(a)   (b)

As tip crosses ML line angle, **transition to mesial root surface** adapting back of tip to mesial root surface. Advance subgingivally and facially using horizontal or slightly oblique strokes until hindered by contact point.

Figure 7.23 # 22 (33) M: (a) ultra-thin straight tip; (b) slim right curved tip

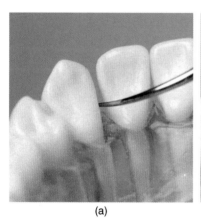
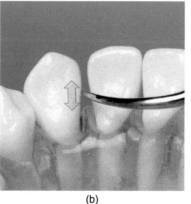

(a)   (b)

Transition *to* mesial interproximal space by keeping back of tip adapted to mesial crown of #22 (FDI 33) while rolling into horizontal adaptation; stroke vertically against mesial surface.

Figure 7.24 #22 (33) M IP: (a) ultra-thin straight tip; (b) slim right curved tip

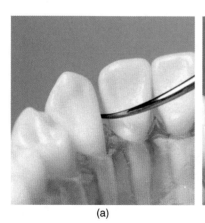
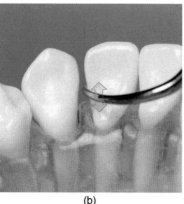

(a)   (b)

Transition to next tooth by adapting face of tip to distal #23 (FDI 32); stroke vertically against the distal surface.

Figure 7.25 #23 (32) D IP: (a) ultra-thin straight tip; (b) slim right curved tip

MODULE 1
ANTERIOR SEXTANT: MANDIBULAR
ANTERIOR LINGUAL

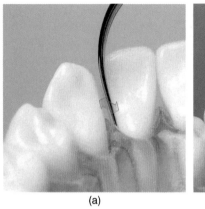
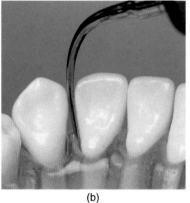

(a)   (b)

Transition *from* **distal interproximal space** to vertical adaptation of the lateral surface. Advance subgingivally and lingually towards DL line angle using horizontal or slightly oblique strokes.

Figure 7.26 #23 (32) D: (a) ultra-thin straight tip; (b) slim right curved tip

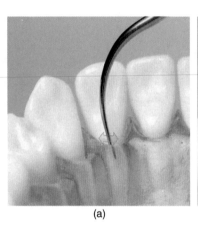
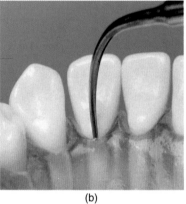

(a)   (b)

Cross the DL line angle of #23 (FDI 32) and proceed with horizontal strokes to advance tip subgingivally and mesially across lingual surface toward ML line angle.

Figure 7.27 #23 (32) L: (a) ultra-thin straight tip; (b) slim right curved tip

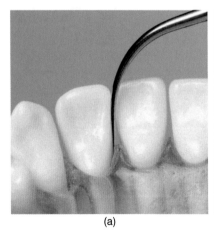
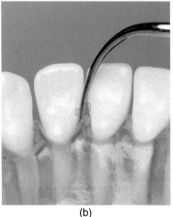

(a)   (b)

As tip crosses ML line angle, maintain vertical adaptation as the back of the tip adapts to the mesial root surface. Stroke horizontally/obliquely, advancing tip subgingivally and facially across surface of mesial root until hindered by contact point.

Figure 7.28 #23 (32) M: (a) ultra-thin straight tip; (b) slim right curved tip

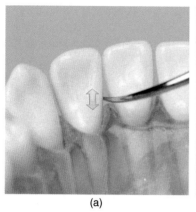 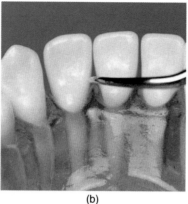

At contact point, transition to horizontal adaptation of the back; stroke tip vertically against mesial surface.

(a)   (b)

Figure 7.29 #23 (32) M IP: (a) ultra-thin straight tip; (b) slim right curved tip

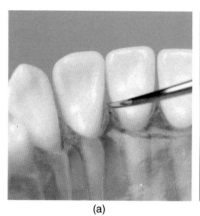 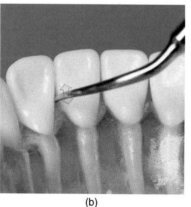

Advance to distal of #24 (FDI 31) by maintaining tip in horizontal orientation and adapting face; stroke vertically against distal surface.

(a)   (b)

Figure 7.30 #24 (31) D IP: (a) ultra-thin straight tip; (b) slim right curved tip

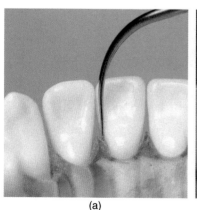 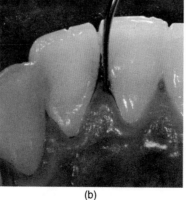

Transition to vertical adaptation of the lateral surface of the tip to the distal surface of #24 (FDI 31). Stroke horizontally/obliquely, advancing tip subgingivally and lingually toward the DL line angle.

(a)   (b)

Figure 7.31 #24 (31) D: (a and b) ultra-thin straight tip

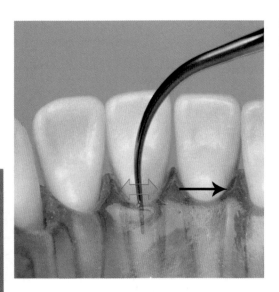

Figure 7.32 #24 (31) L: ultra-thin straight tip. Black arrow indicates repetition of sequence through remainder of sextant

Cross the DL line angle and **proceed through the sextant executing this sequence to completion,** finishing in horizontal orientation on the distal surface of #27 (FDI 43).

Module 2
Posterior Sextant: Maxillary Right Buccal

Table 7.2 Operator position: maxillary right buccal sextant

	Straight tip	Left curved tip
Right-handed		

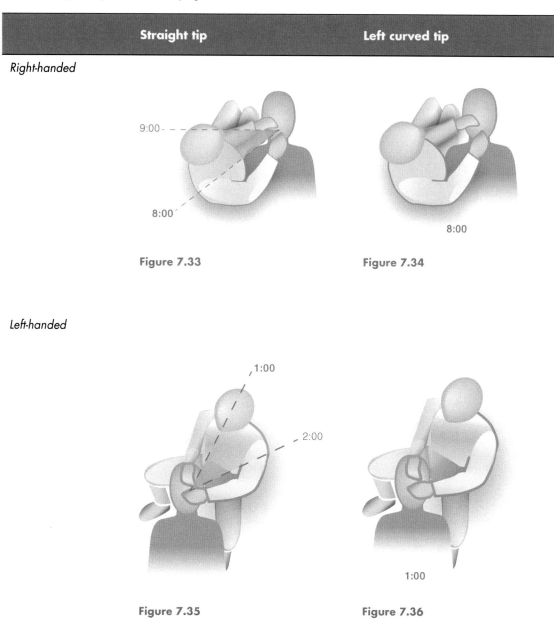

Figure 7.33   **Figure 7.34**

Figure 7.35   **Figure 7.36**

The ideal or recommended operator position is in bold, but can vary to any position within the range stated.

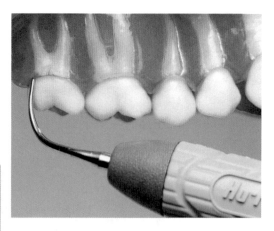

Vertically adapt lateral surface (or back) of active tip at the DB line angle (i.e., point of adaptation) of #2 (FDI 17).

Figure 7.37

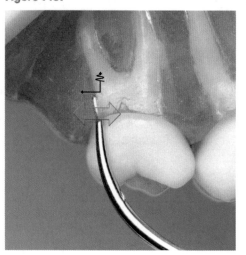

Initiate horizontal strokes to advance tip subgingivally and distally toward the DB line angle.

Figure 7.38 #2 (17) B: standard straight tip; blue arrow indicates direction of the working stroke, black arrows indicate the path of tip advancement from this point

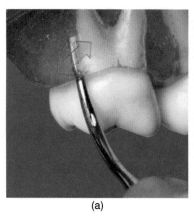
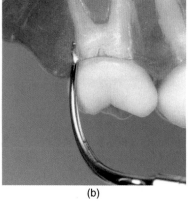

(a)   (b)

As tip crosses DB line angle, **transition to distal root surface** by maintaining vertical adaptation of lateral surface to distal aspect of tooth. Stroke obliquely, advancing tip subgingivally and lingually across the distal root surface.

Figure 7.39 #2 (17) D: (a) standard straight tip; (b) slim left curved tip

ULTRASONIC INSTRUMENTATION TECHNIQUE MODULES

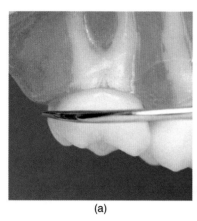
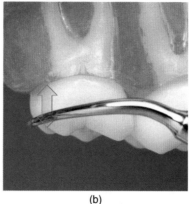

Transition *to* distal interproximal space by horizontally adapting face of tip to distal surface #2 (FDI 17); stroke vertically.

(a)   (b)

Figure 7.40 #2 (17) D IP: (a) standard straight tip; (b) slim left curved tip

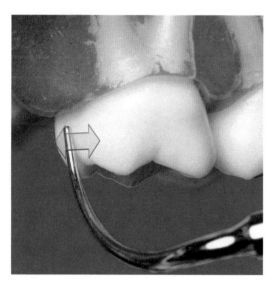

OPTION: As the most posterior tooth does not contact another tooth at the distal aspect, vertical adaptation of the lateral surface can be maintained (instead of transitioning into horizontal adaptation) and the tip stroked horizontally or obliquely across the distal surface of the crown.

Figure 7.41 #2 (17) D IP: slim left curved tip

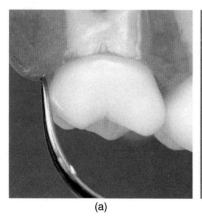
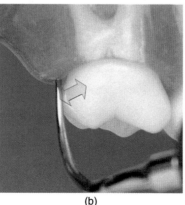

If option offered in Figure 7.41 was not performed, **transition *from* distal interproximal space**, returning to vertical adaptation of the lateral surface; stroke obliquely to retreat tip to DB line angle.

(a)   (b)

Figure 7.42 #2 (17) D: (a) standard straight tip; (b) slim left curved tip

Module 2
POSTERIOR SEXTANT: MAXILLARY
RIGHT BUCCAL

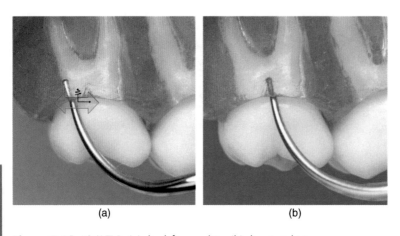

(a)   (b)

As DB line angle is crossed, maintain vertical adaptation of lateral surface and implement horizontal strokes to advance tip subgingivally and mesially across buccal surface.

Figure 7.43 #2 (17) B: (a) slim left curved tip; (b) slim straight tip

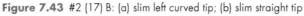

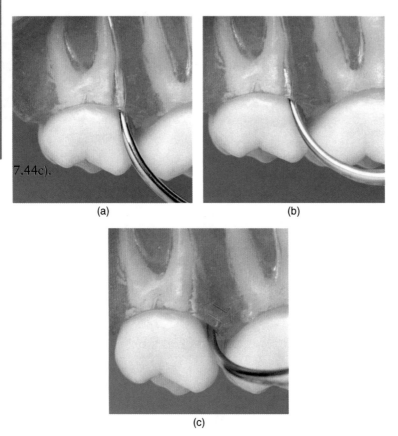

7.44c).

(a)   (b)

(c)

As tip crosses MB line angle, *transition to mesial root surface* by maintaining vertical adaptation as back of tip adapts to mesial surface (Figure 7.44a,b). Stroke obliquely, advancing tip subgingivally and lingually across the mesial root (Figure

Figure 7.44 #2 (17) M: (a) standard straight tip; (b) slim left curved tip; (c) slim left curved tip

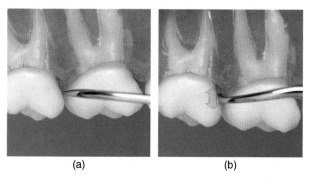

(a)   (b)

Figure 7.45 #2 (17) M IP: (a) standard straight tip; (b) slim left curved tip

Transition *to* mesial interproximal space, keeping back of tip adapted while rolling into horizontal adaptation; stroke vertically against mesial surface #2 (FDI 17).

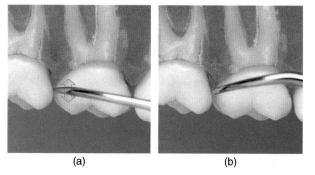

(a)   (b)

Figure 7.46 #3 (16) D IP: (a) standard straight tip; (b) slim left curved tip

Transition to next tooth by adapting face of tip to distal #3 (FDI 16); stroke vertically against the distal surface.

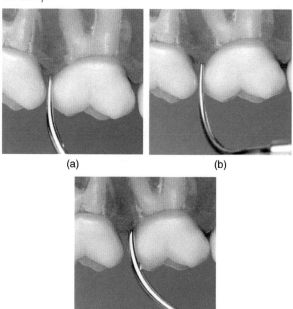

(a)   (b)

(c)

Figure 7.47 #3 (16) D: (a) standard straight tip; (b) slim left curved tip; (c) standard straight tip

Transition *from* distal interproximal space to vertical adaptation of the lateral surface (Figure 7.47a,b). Implement oblique strokes to advance tip subgingivally and facially across distal root surface toward DB line angle (Figure 7.47c).

Module 2
POSTERIOR SEXTANT: MAXILLARY
RIGHT BUCCAL

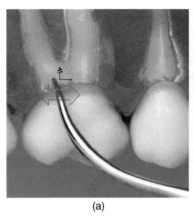
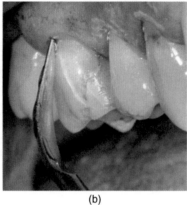

(a)   (b)

As the DB line angle is crossed, maintain vertical adaptation of lateral surface; stroke horizontally, advancing tip subgingivally and mesially across the buccal surface of #3 (FDI 16).

Figure 7.48 #3 (16) B: Standard straight tips from two different manufacturers (a,b)

Box 7.3: Technique pointer: Early furcation involvement

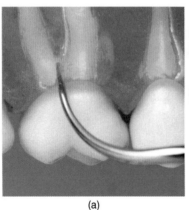
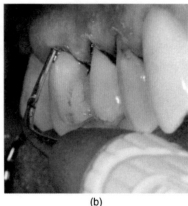

(a)   (b)

As the pocket is suprabony and has not entered the furcation, instrumentation of a Grade I furcation defect is performed as the furcation is encountered within the instrumentation sequence: buccal and lingual furcations treated as encountered during instrumentation of the buccal and lingual surfaces; mesial and distal furcations treated as encountered during instrumentation of the interproximal surfaces.

Figure 7.49 #3(16) B furcation: (a) slim left curved tip; (b) from clinician's perspective

Instrumentation of more involved furcations (Grades II–IV) requires a furcation-specific technique and sequence, which is presented in the Advanced Furcation Defects Module.

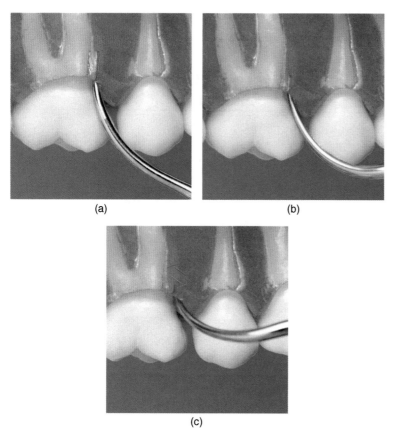

As tip crosses MB line angle, maintain vertical adaptation as the back of the tip adapts to the mesial root surface (Figure 7.50a,b). Stroke obliquely, advancing tip subgingivally and lingually across the mesial root surface (Figure 7.50c).

(a)   (b)

(c)

Figure 7.50 #3 (16) M: (a) standard straight tip; (b) slim left curved tip; (c) slim left curved tip

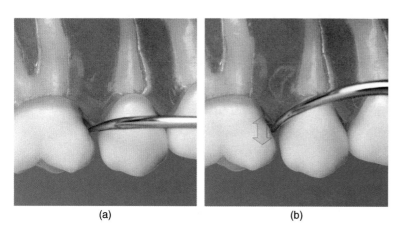

Move into the interproximal space, transitioning to horizontal adaptation of the back of the tip; stroke vertically against mesial surface #3 (FDI 16).

(a)   (b)

Figure 7.51 #3 (16) M IP: (a) standard straight tip; (b) slim left curved tip

Module 2
POSTERIOR SEXTANT: MAXILLARY
RIGHT BUCCAL

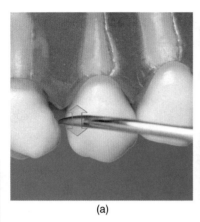 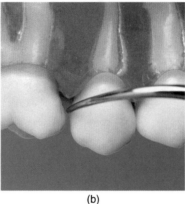

Advance to distal of #4 (FDI 15) by maintaining horizontal orientation and adapting face of tip; stroke vertically against distal surface.

(a)   (b)

Figure 7.52 #4 (15) D IP: (a) standard straight tip; (b) slim left curved tip

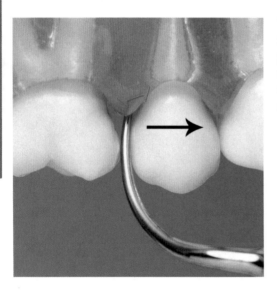

Transition to vertical adaptation of the lateral surface of the tip. Stroke obliquely to advance tip subgingivally and facially toward DB line angle. **Proceed through the sextant executing the sequence to completion,** ending in horizontal orientation on the mesial surface of #5 (FDI 14).

Figure 7.53 #4 (15) D: slim left curved tip. Black arrow indicates repetition of sequence through remainder of sextant

Box 7.4: Supplemental instrumentation of interproximal space

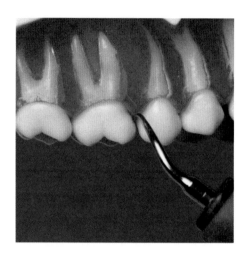

Figure 7.54 In the maxillary right buccal sextant, the right curved tip is used with oblique adaptation to supplement instrumentation of the interproximal space

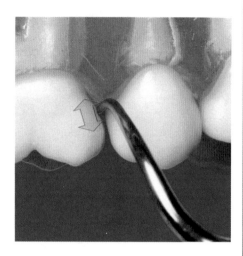

Figure 7.55 # 3(16) M IP: slim right curved tip. Note oblique adaptation of lateral surface

A supplemental approach to scaling calculus from the interproximal space utilizes the "other" curved tip in traditional oblique adaptation. Remember that the curved tips are a complementary and site-specific pair; the "other" tip being the curved tip which is not indicated for that particular treatment site. For example, in the maxillary right buccal sextant, the RIGHT curved tip is utilized in this supplemental approach (Figure 7.54) instead of the recommended LEFT curved tip. A lateral surface of the right curved tip is *obliquely* adapted to a mesial (Figure 7.55) or distal surface and stroked vertically.

This approach should be used only as a supplement to, and not a replacement for, the primary vertical technique. As an example of how to efficiently incorporate this supplemental technique into the primary sequence, we will look at the maxillary right quadrant again. After completing primary instrumentation from the buccal perspective using the LEFT curved tip, debride the palatal interproximal spaces using the supplemental technique before switching to the RIGHT curved tip. With the RIGHT curved tip in place, perform the primary sequence on all palatal surfaces, then return to the buccal to supplement debridement of the interproximal surfaces.

All other sextants

The systematic approach to instrumentation practiced in Modules 1 and 2 can be readily applied in any area of the dentition from the operator positions recommended in Tables 7.3 and 7.4. Compared to hand instrumentation, which requires multiple changes in operator position to accommodate access and leverage, all ultrasonic instrumentation can typically be implemented from just two operator positions, assuming the patient's head is suitably turned.

Table 7.3 Operator positions: right-handed clinicians

Operator position	Sextant
8:00 (8:00–9:00) 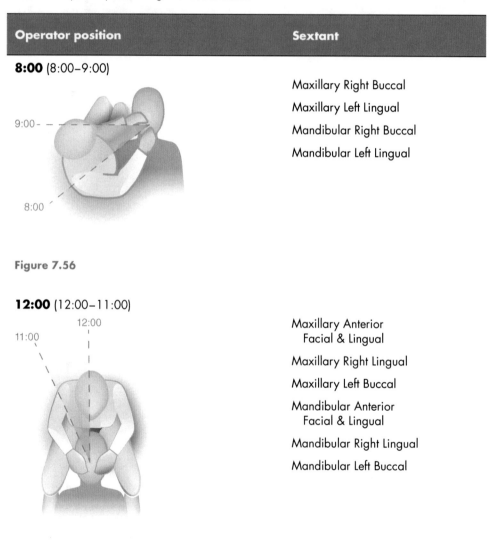	Maxillary Right Buccal Maxillary Left Lingual Mandibular Right Buccal Mandibular Left Lingual

Figure 7.56

12:00 (12:00–11:00)	Maxillary Anterior Facial & Lingual Maxillary Right Lingual Maxillary Left Buccal Mandibular Anterior Facial & Lingual Mandibular Right Lingual Mandibular Left Buccal

Figure 7.57

The ideal or recommended operator position is in bold, but can vary to any position within the range stated.

Table 7.4 Operator positions: left-handed clinicians

Operator position	Sextant
12:00 (12:00–1:00)	

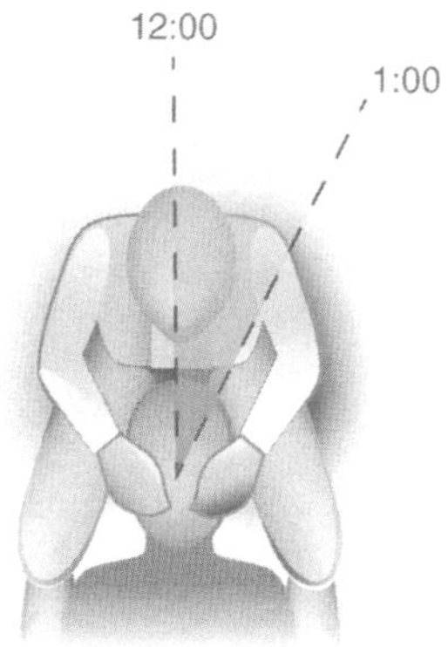

Maxillary Anterior
  Facial & Lingual
Maxillary Right Buccal

Maxillary Left Lingual

Mandibular Anterior
  Facial & Lingual

Mandibular Right Buccal

Mandibular Left Lingual

Figure 7.58

4:00 (4:00–3:00)

Maxillary Left Buccal

Maxillary Right Lingual

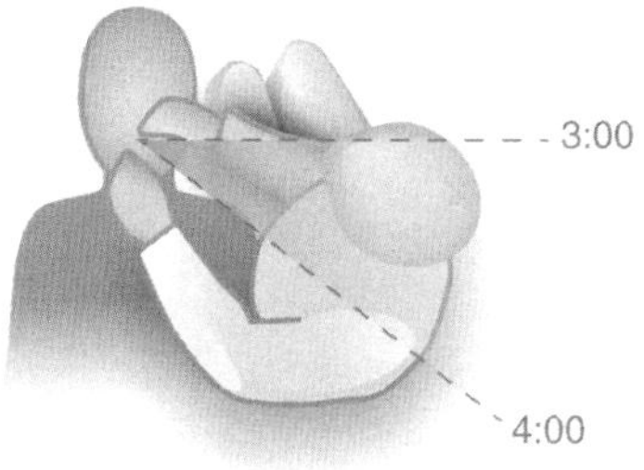

Mandibular Left Buccal

Mandibular Right Lingual

Figure 7.59

The ideal or recommended operator position is in bold, but can vary to any position within the range stated.

ULTRASONIC INSTRUMENTATION
TECHNIQUE MODULES

ADVANCED FURCATION DEFECTS (GRADES II–IV) INSTRUMENTATION MODULES

The complexity of furcation anatomy makes predictable and effective instrumentation of the involved surfaces difficult. Buccal and lingual Grade II furcation defects can be treated effectively by nonsurgical ultrasonic therapy (Del Peloso Ribeiro et al., 2006, 2007), while Grade II interproximal furcation involvements respond less favorably by comparison (Del Peloso Ribeiro et al., 2007). In more advanced furcational defects, nonsurgical therapy is frequently ineffective as diminished access compromises the ability to perform adequate instrumentation (Ammons and Harrington, 2002). Whether intervention is surgical or nonsurgical, a focused effort and a modified technique are required to navigate the ultrasonic tip through the complex furcation morphology in a manner that both optimizes deposit removal and minimizes root surface alteration.

Furcation-specific, ball-end tips (Figure 7.60) are highly preferred for furcation instrumentation, as the spherical tip not only conforms

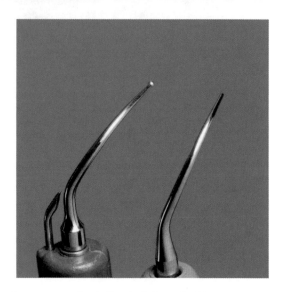

Figure 7.61 The ball-end of the right furcation tip compared to the pointed end of the right curved tip

better to the predominantly concave contours of the furcations, but also eliminates the risk of inadvertent root gouging by a pointed tip, thereby easing and improving accessibility to all aspects of the furcation (Oda and Ishikawa, 1989; Takacs et al., 1993). However, the limited utilization of these ball-end tips in practice (low sales resulted in a major manufacturer

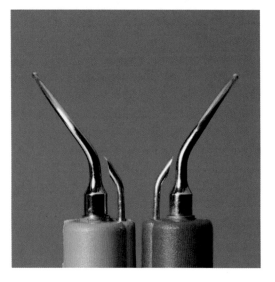

Figure 7.60 Furcation-specific ball-end tips, left and right curved

Table 7.5 Furcation tip designs: indications for use

Tip configuration	Location of furcation
Right furcation ball tip or Left curved tip	Maxillary right buccal Maxillary left lingual Mandibular left buccal Mandibular right lingual
Left furcation ball tip or Right curved tip	Maxillary right lingual Maxillary left buccal Mandibular left lingual Mandibular right buccal

discontinuing production in 2012) indicates the more common use of the pointed curved tips instead (Figure 7.61). This is a concern, as use of the left/right curved tips is less effective in furcations (Takacs et al., 1993) and increases the likelihood for inadvertent root surface damage during furcation debridement.

That said, instructional modules for both the furcation ball and pointed curved tips are provided. Each module assumes use of the proper tip configuration (left or right, Table 7.5) and operator position (Tables 7.3 and 7.4) for the furcation to be treated. Although the sequences delineated for the left/right pointed curved tips include modifications (to the primary instrumentation sequence) intended to avoid contact of the point of the tip to the root structure, the ability to safely and effectively adapt the pointed curved tips in advanced furcations, closed or open, is limited.

Furcation Module 1
Buccal / Lingual Furcations: Curved Tip

FURCATION EXEMPLIFIED: BUCCAL FURCATION
                          #3 (FDI 16)
TIP DESIGN UTILIZED: *LEFT CURVED*

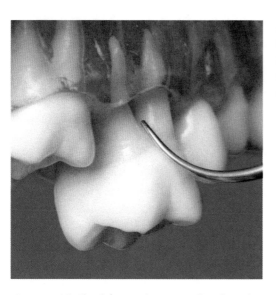

Adapt active area of back of tip (preferred for concave anatomy) or lateral surface to entrance of furcation. Debride entrance using a series of short, overlapping horizontal or oblique strokes while advancing tip into the dome of the furcation.

Figure 7.62 Slim left curved tip vertically adapted at entrance of buccal furcation #3 (16)

FURCATION MODULE 1
BUCCAL / LINGUAL FURCATIONS:
CURVED TIP

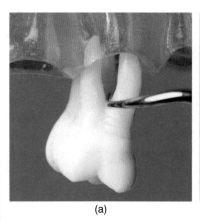
(a)

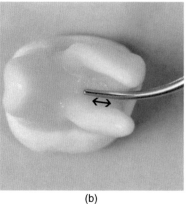
(b)

While maintaining adaptation of active surface of tip at 0 degrees angulation to the dome, debride the dome with short, in-and-out strokes.

Figure 7.63 #3 (16) dome of buccal furcation: (a) buccal perspective, note 0° angulation to dome; (b) apical perspective. Black arrow indicates direction of working stroke

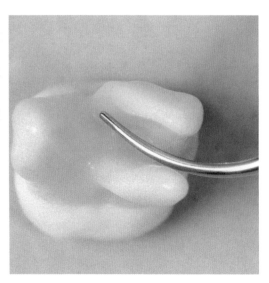

In maxillary molar furcations, take care to prevent point of tip from contacting palatal root, if exposed, during debridement of the dome. When possible, angle the tip to pass between the palatal and mesial or distal roots.

Figure 7.64 # 3(16) dome of buccal furcation: angling of the left curved tip to pass between palatal and mesial roots

ULTRASONIC INSTRUMENTATION TECHNIQUE MODULES

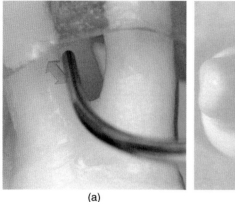 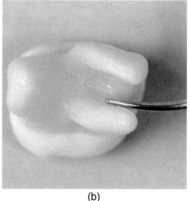

(a)   (b)

From the dome, adapt the back of the tip horizontally against the internal surface of the distal root[1]. Maintaining horizontal adaptation, stroke the back vertically (up/down) over the internal surface of the distal root.

Figure 7.65 # 3(16) buccal furcation, internal surface of distal root: (a) buccal perspective; (b) apical perspective

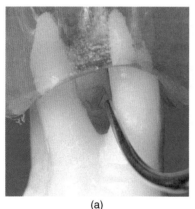 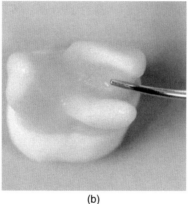

(a)   (b)

Retreat tip to dome and roll slightly to adapt the lateral surface of the active area horizontal to the internal surface of the mesial root.[2] Maintaining this horizontal orientation, stroke the lateral surface vertically over the internal surface of the mesial root.

Figure 7.66 #3 (16) buccal furcation, internal surface of mesial root: (a) buccal perspective; (b) apical perspective

FURCATION MODULE 1
BUCCAL / LINGUAL FURCATIONS:
CURVED TIP

---

[1] If the lateral tip surface is adapted to the dome, the back of the tip is already horizontally oriented to the distal root; if the back of the tip is adapted to the dome, slightly roll tip to orient the back towards the distal root.

[2] The ideal surface to adapt to the deeply concave internal mesial root surface is the convex back of the curved tip; but, from the buccal aspect, the back cannot be readily adapted in most situations. However, from the palatal aspect, the back of the tip is more adaptable to the internal surface of the mesial root. Therefore, when accessible, debridement of the internal surface of the mesial root should be accomplished primarily from the palatal aspect.

Box 7.5: Technique pointer: Furcation debridement

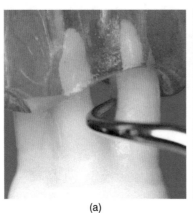

(a)

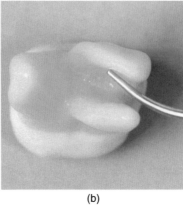

(b)

While it may seem rationale to utilize the face of the tip to debride the internal surface of the mesial root (Figure 7.67a), adaptation of the face is contraindicated because it inherently results in the point of the tip contacting the root structure and causing root gouging (Figure 7.67b).

Figure 7.67 #3 (16) buccal furcation, internal surface of mesial root: (a) buccal perspective showing adaptation of the face to the mesial root; (b) apical perspective showing point gouging internal surface of mesial root when face of tip is adapted

Furcation Module 2
Buccal / Lingual Furcations: Ball Tip

FURCATION EXEMPLIFIED: BUCCAL FURCATION
                        #3 (FDI 16)
TIP DESIGN UTILIZED: *RIGHT FURCATION BALL*

As designated in Table 7.5, the recommended furcation ball tip configuration (left or right) for any area is the opposite of the configuration recommended for using pointed curved tips. For example, in this maxillary right buccal quadrant, the RIGHT furcation tip is indicated instead of the LEFT curved tip. However, because the active area of these tips is spherical in shape, either configuration (left or right) may be used in any area as determined by anatomy and access, and in some furcations, use of both configurations may be needed to accomplish thorough debridement. Regardless of the tip configuration used, the instrumentation technique and sequence executed remains the same.

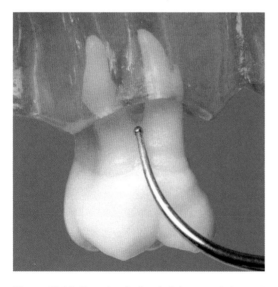

Vertically adapt either the back or lateral surface of the sphere to the entrance of the furcation. Debride entrance using a series of short, overlapping horizontal and vertical strokes while advancing tip into the dome of the furcation.

Figure 7.68 Furcation ball-end right curved tip vertically adapted at entrance of buccal furcation #3 (16)

FURCATION MODULE 2
BUCCAL / LINGUAL FURCATIONS:
BALL TIP

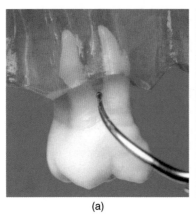 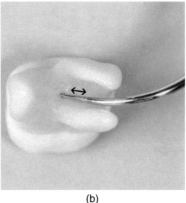

(a)   (b)

Figure 7.69 #3 (16) dome of buccal furcation: (a) buccal perspective; (b) apical perspective. Black arrow indicates direction of working stroke

Maintaining adaptation of the sphere to the dome, debride the dome with short, in-and-out strokes.

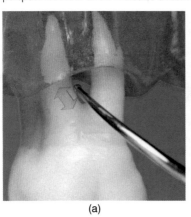 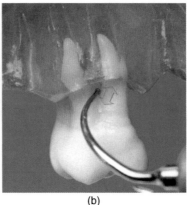

(a)   (b)

Figure 7.70 #3 (16) buccal furcation: (a) internal surface of distal root; (b) internal surface of mesial buccal root

From the dome, stroke the sphere vertically (up/down) over the internal surfaces of the distal (Figure 7.70a) and mesial (Figure 7.70b) roots.

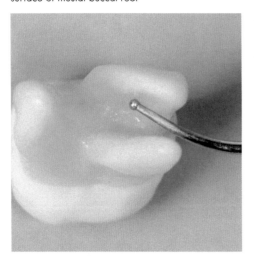

Figure 7.71 #3 (16) buccal furcation: apical perspective showing adaptation of convex sphere to concavity of internal surface of mesial buccal root

The face of the tip can be adapted towards the mesial root to improve contact of the convex sphere with the concave internal surface, optimizing debridement without concern for root gouging (contrast with Figure 7.67b).

ULTRASONIC INSTRUMENTATION TECHNIQUE MODULES

Furcation Module 3
Mesial Furcations: Curved Tip

FURCATION EXEMPLIFIED: MESIAL FURCATION #3 (FDI 16)
                                    PALATAL ACCESS
TIP DESIGN UTILIZED: *RIGHT CURVED*

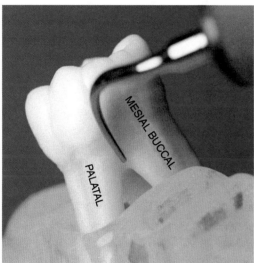

Vertically adapt active area of lateral surface to the entrance of mesial furcation. Debride entrance using a series of short, overlapping horizontal or oblique strokes while advancing lateral surface into the dome of the furcation.

Figure 7.72 Slim right curved tip adapted at entrance of mesial furcation #3 (16)

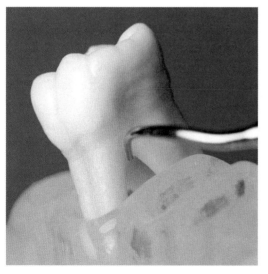

While maintaining adaptation of lateral surface of tip at 0° angulation to the dome, debride the dome with short, in-and-out strokes.

Figure 7.73 #3 (16)
dome of mesial furcation; note 0° angulation to the dome

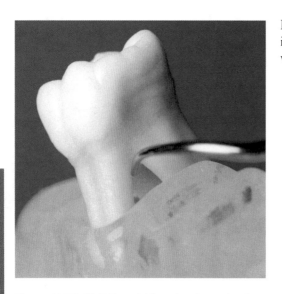

Figure 7.74 #3 (16) mesial furcation: internal surface of palatal root

From the dome, stroke the back of the tip against the internal surface of the palatal root in an oblique or vertical pattern.

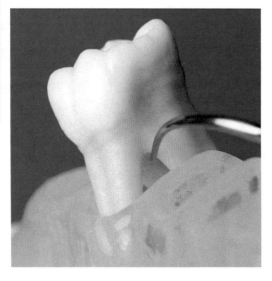

Figure 7.75 #3 (16) mesial furcation: internal surface of mesial buccal root

Retreat tip to dome to adapt the lateral surface to the internal surface of the mesial buccal root and stroke vertically. Avoid adapting the face of the tip to the internal surface of the mesial buccal root because of the inadequate contact between the two concave surfaces and likelihood of the point engaging the root surface.

Furcation Module 4
Mesial Furcations: Ball Tip

FURCATION EXEMPLIFIED: MESIAL FURCATION #3 (FDI 16)
                          PALATAL ACCESS
TIP DESIGN UTILIZED: *LEFT FURCATION BALL*

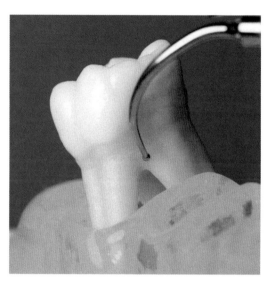

Vertically adapt either the back or lateral surface of the sphere to the entrance of furcation. Debride entrance using a series of short, overlapping horizontal and vertical strokes while advancing tip into the dome of the furcation.

Figure 7.76 Furcation ball-end left curved tip adapted at entrance of mesial furcation #3 (16)

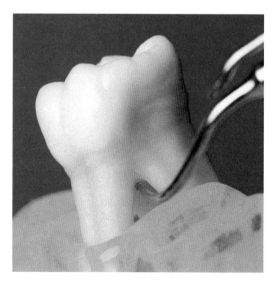

Maintaining adaptation of the sphere to the dome, debride the dome with short, in-and-out strokes.

Figure 7.77 #3 (16) dome of mesial furcation

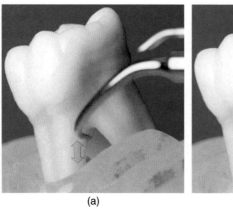 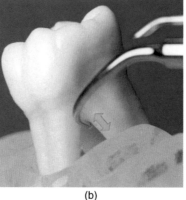

From the dome, stroke the sphere vertically (up/down) over the internal surfaces of the palatal (Figure 7.78a) and mesial buccal (Figure 7.78b) roots.

(a)   (b)

Figure 7.78 #3 (16) mesial furcation: (a) internal surface of palatal root; (b) internal surface of mesial buccal root

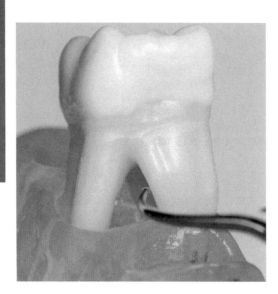

Specific to the mesial buccal root, roll the face of the tip towards the mesial buccal root to readily adapt the convex sphere to the concavity of the internal root surface for optimal debridement without concern for gouging.

Figure 7.79 #3 (16) mesial furcation: adaptation of face of tip to mesial buccal root facilitates contact of convex sphere to concavity of internal root surface

Furcation Module 5
Distal Furcations: Curved & Ball Tips

FURCATION EXEMPLIFIED: DISTAL FURCATION #3 (FDI 16)
                                    BUCCAL ACCESS
TIP DESIGN UTILIZED: *LEFT CURVED*

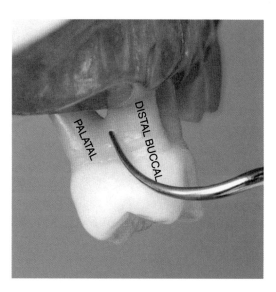

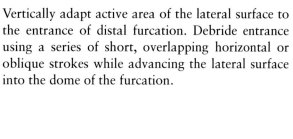

Vertically adapt active area of the lateral surface to the entrance of distal furcation. Debride entrance using a series of short, overlapping horizontal or oblique strokes while advancing the lateral surface into the dome of the furcation.

Figure 7.80 Slim left curved tip vertically adapted at entrance of distal furcation #3 (16)

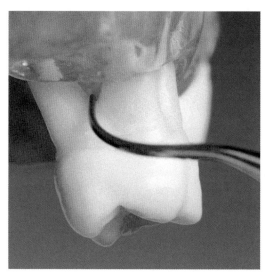

With lateral surface of tip adapted at 0° angulation to the dome, debride the dome with short, in-and-out strokes.

Figure 7.81 #3 (16) dome of distal furcation

FURCATION MODULE 5
DISTAL FURCATIONS: CURVED & BALL TIPS

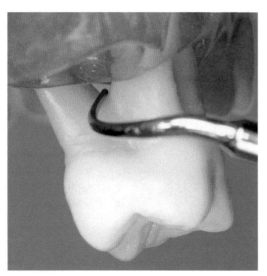

From the dome, stroke the back of the tip against the internal surface of the palatal root in an oblique or vertical pattern.

Figure 7.82 #3(16) distal furcation: internal surface of palatal root

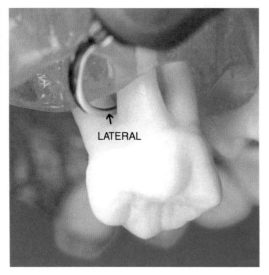

Retreat tip to dome to adapt the lateral surface to the internal surface of the distal root and stroke vertically. Avoid adapting the face of the tip to the internal surface of the distal root because of the likelihood of the point engaging the root surface.

Figure 7.83 #3 (16) distal furcation: internal surface of distal buccal root

FURCATION EXEMPLIFIED: DISTAL FURCATION #3 (FDI 16)
                         BUCCAL ACCESS
TIP DESIGN UTILIZED: *RIGHT FURCATION BALL*

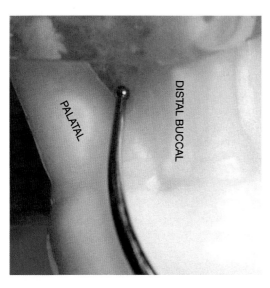

PALATAL

DISTAL BUCCAL

Figure 7.84 Right furcation ball tip adapted at entrance of distal furcation #3 (16)

Instrumentation of the distal furcation using a furcation ball tip follows the same sequence as the left curved tip, but modified in adaptation to optimize contact of the sphere, as previously described for buccal and mesial furcations. Select tip configuration (left or right) based on access (buccal or palatal) and anatomy. In the furcation exemplified here (#3D (FDI 16) accessed from the buccal), the RIGHT furcation ball tip is utilized.

FURCATION MODULE 5
DISTAL FURCATIONS: CURVED & BALL TIPS

IMPLANT AND SUPRAGINGIVAL INSTRUMENTATION

Implant instrumentation technique

The selection of a tip design appropriate for implant debridement is discussed in Chapters 2 and 4. Regardless of the design of the tip utilized, effective ultrasonic debridement of a dental implant mimics ultrasonic debridement of a natural tooth in both the technique employed and sequence followed.

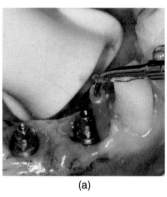 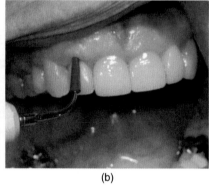

(a)   (b)

With tip vertically adapted, implement appropriate ultrasonic stroking and transitional sequences to advance across all surfaces of the implant.

Figure 7.85 Ideal vertical adaptation of implant-specific tip to (a) unrestored and (b) restored abutments (Image (b) courtesy of Lisa Copeland, RDH)

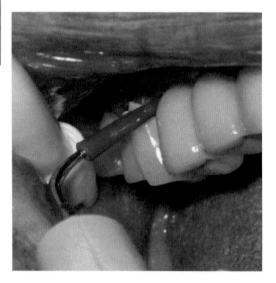

Depending on the contours of the restoration, it may not be possible to access all implant surfaces and still maintain angulation at 0–15°. Use of a plastic or carbon fiber implant-specific tip allows for a greater range of angulation between the tip and the implant surface, facilitating access without the risk of severely damaging the implant (Unursaikhan et al., 2012).

Figure 7.86 Modified adaptation of a plastic implant-specific tip to an abutment with a highly contoured restoration. This angulation is needed to access the subgingival space, but only acceptable when a plastic or carbon fiber implant-specific tip is utilized. (Image courtesy of Lisa Copeland, RDH)

ULTRASONIC INSTRUMENTATION TECHNIQUE MODULES

Supragingival instrumentation technique

Performing thorough ultrasonic scaling and debridement of supragingival deposits is much easier than subgingival instrumentation because adaptation, angulation, and stroking of the ultrasonic tip are not confined by surrounding tissues, and the clinician has direct visibility of the treatment surface.

While it may be intuitive for the clinician to implement supragingival instrumentation using a traditional oblique approach, these authors recommend utilization of the vertical approach for all of the reasons outlined in Chapter 6, Section 6.1. Selection of tip design and power setting appropriate for the type of deposit and anatomy are assumed.

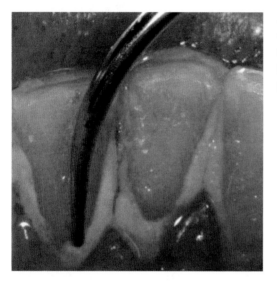

Adapt tip vertically at any edge of the supragingival deposit. Implement appropriate stroking and transitional sequences to advance tip across all coronal surfaces until visually and tactilely free of supragingival deposits.

Figure 7.87 #23 (32) L: standard straight tip vertically adapted at edge of supragingival deposit

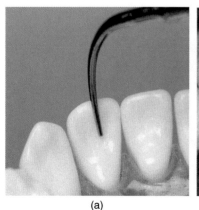
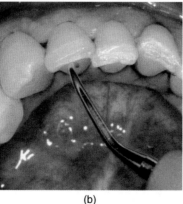

As direct access and vertical adaptation ease utilization of any surface of the tip, the convex back can be adapted to the lingual concavities of coronal surfaces to improve conformity and increase the efficiency of deposit removal.

(a)   (b)

Figure 7.88 #23 (32) L: convex back of the slim right curved tip vertically adapted to convex surface of the lingual fossa; (a) lingual view, (b) occlusal view

REFERENCES

Ammons WF and Harrington GW. Furcation: the problem and its management. In: Carranza's Clinical Periodontology, (eds.) Newman MG, Takei HH, Carranza FA. 9th edn. Philadelphia: W.B. Saunders; 2002.

Del Peloso Ribeiro E, Bittencourt S, Ambrosano GM, Nociti FH Jr, Sallum EA, Sallum AW et al. Povidone-iodine used as an adjunct to non-surgical treatment of furcation involvements. *J Periodontol* 2006; 77: 211–7.

Del Peloso Ribeiro E, Bittencourt S, Nociti FH Jr, Sallum EA, Sallum AW, Casati MZ. Comparative study of ultrasonic instrumentation for the non-surgical treatment of interproximal and non-interproximal furcation involvements. *J Periodontol* 2007; 78: 224–30.

Oda S, Ishikawa I. In vitro effectiveness of a newly-designed ultrasonic scaler tip for furcation areas. *J Periodontol* 1989; 60: 634–9.

Takacs VJ, Tryggve L, Perala DG, Adams DF. Efficacy of 5 machining instruments in scaling of molar furcations. *J Periodontol* 1993; 64: 228–36.

Unursaikhan O, Lee JS, Cha JK, Park JC, Jung UW, Kim CS et al. Comparative evaluation of roughness of titanium surfaces treated by different hygiene instruments. *J Periodontal Implant Sci* 2012; 42: 88–94.

ULTRASONIC INSTRUMENTATION TECHNIQUE MODULES

Chapter 8

Case studies in ultrasonic debridement

CHAPTER OBJECTIVE

Through the presentation of clinical cases, this chapter integrates the content addressed in preceding chapters and demonstrates the application of evidence-based theory to case-based decision making in the clinical practice of periodontics.

CASE A: INITIAL AND SUPPORTIVE PERIODONTAL THERAPY

Presentation

This 53-year-old Caucasian male presented to a general dental practice for a dental examination and subsequent care after not receiving any dental care since at least seven years prior, due to financial constraints. The patient suggested that his spouse compelled him to make an appointment as she was concerned with the appearance of his teeth.

Medical history

- The patient's height and weight are 5′ 7″ (1.70 m) and 190 lbs (86.2 kg). Body mass index (BMI) = 29.8.

- The patient has smoked cigarettes since the age of 17, and is currently smoking an average of a half a pack (10 cigarettes) per day.

- Three years ago, the patient was diagnosed with high blood pressure and was prescribed valsartan, an angiotensin receptor blocker, 160 mg/daily.

- The patient's blood pressure control has improved and is now averaging 133/80 mm Hg. He reportedly is reevaluated by his physician every three months.

Clinical examination

- Moderate–heavy supragingival and subgingival calcified deposits at multiple sites.

- Soft tissue changes (contour and color changes) consistent with inflammation were noted at multiple sites, especially at posterior lingual and palatal sextants.

- Generalized bleeding upon probing was noted.

- Carious enamel and root surfaces were noted at multiple teeth.

- Exposed root surface structure was noted at multiple teeth.

- Broken restoration noted at tooth #30 (FDI 46).

Ultrasonic Periodontal Debridement: Theory and Technique, First Edition. Marie D. George, Timothy G. Donley and Philip M. Preshaw.
© 2014 John Wiley & Sons, Inc. Published 2014 by John Wiley & Sons, Inc.

Initial Therapy Patient
Pre-treatment Photos

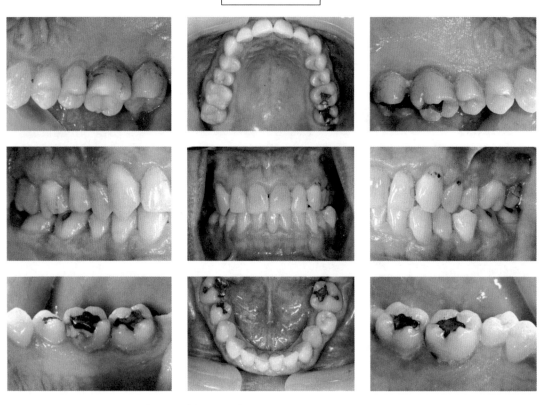

Figure 8.1 Pretreatment intraoral views of the initial therapy patient

- Malocclusion of left posterior with crowding and challenging oral hygiene access.

Radiographic examination

- Moderate bone loss with a vertical component was noted at teeth #2–3 (FDI 17, 16), 14–15 (FDI 26, 27) and distal to tooth #18 (FDI 37). Other posterior areas of mild horizontal bone loss were noted.

- Subgingival calculus deposits were noted interproximally at most teeth and distal to all second molars.

- Mesial root concavity was noted at tooth #5 (FDI 14).

Risk assessment and diagnosis

- Periodontal risk factors included tobacco use, lack of regular care and overweight (BMI of 29.8 places this patient in the overweight category).

- Diagnosis: Chronic periodontitis with isolated areas of slight to moderate loss of periodontal support.

- The lack of more generalized and advanced loss of periodontal support despite the patient's risk factors, lack of previous care, and generalized heavy etiology was noteworthy.

PERIO CHART

Patient Name: Initial Periodontal Therapy Patient
Patient ID:
Exam Date: Baseline examination

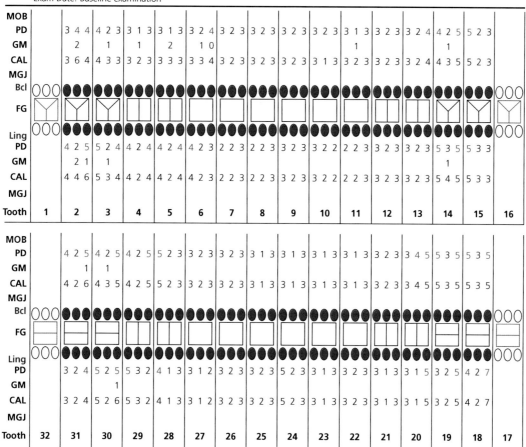

Maxillary (teeth 1–16) — Buccal

	1	2	3	4	5	6	7	8	9	10	11	12	13	14	15	16
MOB																
PD		3 4 4	4 2 3	3 1 3	3 1 3	3 2 4	3 2 3	3 2 3	3 2 3	3 2 3	3 1 3	3 2 3	3 2 4	4 2 5	5 2 3	
GM		2	1	1	2	1 0						1		1		
CAL		3 6 4	4 3 3	3 2 3	3 3 3	3 3 4	3 2 3	3 2 3	3 2 3	3 1 3	3 2 3	3 2 3	3 2 4	4 3 5	5 2 3	
MGJ																

Maxillary (teeth 1–16) — Lingual

	1	2	3	4	5	6	7	8	9	10	11	12	13	14	15	16
MGJ																
PD		4 2 5	5 2 4	4 2 4	4 2 4	4 2 3	2 2 3	2 2 3	3 2 3	3 2 2	2 2 3	3 2 3	3 2 3	5 3 5	5 3 3	
GM		2 1	1											1		
CAL		4 4 6	5 3 4	4 2 4	4 2 4	4 2 3	2 2 3	2 2 3	3 2 3	3 2 2	2 2 3	3 2 3	3 2 3	5 4 5	5 3 3	
MGJ																
Tooth	1	2	3	4	5	6	7	8	9	10	11	12	13	14	15	16

Mandibular (teeth 32–17) — Buccal

	32	31	30	29	28	27	26	25	24	23	22	21	20	19	18	17
MOB																
PD		4 2 5	4 2 5	4 2 5	5 2 3	3 2 3	3 2 3	3 1 3	3 1 3	3 1 3	3 1 3	3 2 3	3 4 5	5 3 5	5 3 5	
GM		1	1													
CAL		4 2 6	4 3 5	4 2 5	5 2 3	3 2 3	3 2 3	3 1 3	3 1 3	3 1 3	3 1 3	3 2 3	3 4 5	5 3 5	5 3 5	
MGJ																

Mandibular (teeth 32–17) — Lingual

	32	31	30	29	28	27	26	25	24	23	22	21	20	19	18	17
MGJ																
PD		3 2 4	5 2 5	5 3 2	4 1 3	3 1 2	3 2 3	3 2 3	5 2 3	3 1 3	3 2 3	3 1 3	3 1 5	3 2 5	4 2 7	
GM			1													
CAL		3 2 4	5 2 6	5 3 2	4 1 3	3 1 2	3 2 3	3 2 3	5 2 3	3 1 3	3 2 3	3 1 3	3 1 5	3 2 5	4 2 7	
MGJ																
Tooth	32	31	30	29	28	27	26	25	24	23	22	21	20	19	18	17

Figure 8.2 Baseline periodontal charting of the initial therapy patient

Initial Therapy Patient
Baseline FMX

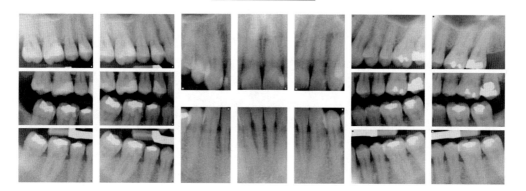

Figure 8.3 Baseline radiographs of the initial therapy patient

Treatment planned

- Full mouth nonsurgical periodontal debridement scheduled over two sessions
- Crown – porcelain/ceramic substrate #3 (FDI 16), #5 (FDI 14), #15 (FDI 27), and #30 (FDI 46)

Periodontal treatment provided

Session 1:

- Initial ultrasonic debridement of maxillary right, mandibular right, and mandibular anterior sextants.
  - 36 mg 2% lidocaine w/0.018 mg epinephrine administered via IANB
  - 72 mg 4% articaine w/0.009 mg epinephrine administered via infiltration

Session 2:

- Initial ultrasonic debridement of maxillary anterior, maxillary left, and mandibular left sextants
- Supportive ultrasonic debridement of sextants previously treated at Session 1

- 36 mg 2% lidocaine w/0.018 mg epinephrine administered via IANB on the left
- 85 mg of a commercially-available 2.5% lidocaine/2.5% prilocaine anesthetic gel applied subgingivally to maxillary sextants

Discussion

Although the intent was to complete the initial debridement therapy in two sessions scheduled one week apart, the patient failed to show for the second appointment. Numerous attempts were made to reschedule him in a timely manner, but scheduling conflicts delayed the second session by three months. By then, reevaluation and supportive maintenance therapy in the sextants previously treated were indicated, and therefore, completed during the same appointment.

A. INITIAL THERAPY

The presence of moderate–heavy calculus deposits required that initial debridement therapy be implemented in two stages. A standard diameter tip, straight by default and with one-bend, was utilized first, at a medium–high power setting, to reduce the calculus deposits to a lesser degree in both anterior (Figure 8.4) and posterior areas (Figure 8.5).

As the clinician is right-handed, scaling of the mandibular anterior lingual sextant

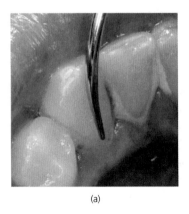 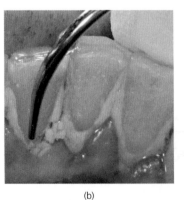 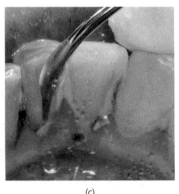

(a) (b) (c)

Figure 8.4 Standard diameter cylindrical tip vertically adapted at 0° angulation to the lingual surfaces of (a) #22 (FDI 33); (b) #24 (FDI 31); and (c) #25 (FDI 41)

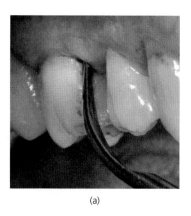 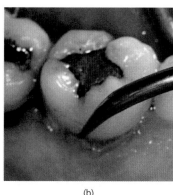 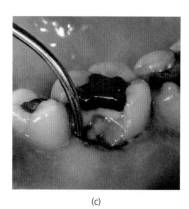

(a)   (b)   (c)

Figure 8.5 (a) Proper adaptation of rectangular standard tip to #3M (FDI 16); (b) tapping the point of the tip against heavy calculus at the gingival margin of #19L (FDI 36); (c) appropriate adaptation and advancement into the pocket at #30ML (FDI 46)

commenced at the midline of #22 (FDI 33) (Figure 8.4a) and continued, following the transitional sequence, to the distal of #27 (FDI 43). Removal/reduction of the heavy supragingival calculus preceded subgingival scaling and occurred as the oscillating tip engaged with the edges of the supragingival deposits (Figure 8.4b,c)

Scaling of various posterior sextants is illustrated in Figure 8.5a–c. The rectangular standard tip utilized in the maxillary right buccal (Figure 8.5a) and mandibular left lingual (Figure 8.5b) sextants provided greater force against the heavy calculus deposits (without increasing the power setting), compared to the cylindrical standard tip utilized to scale the fractured surface in the mandibular right lingual sextant (Figure 8.5c). A tapping stroke (Figure 8.5b) was utilized to break up the heavy calculus deposits at the lingual gingival margins of the mandibular molar prior to initiating subgingival instrumentation.

Figure 8.6 illustrates implementation of the transitional sequence used to advance the tip, as described in Chapter 7, during scaling of the mandibular right buccal sextant.

On removal or reduction of the calculus deposits in the posterior and anterior sextants, the clinician switched to slim

diameter tips and appropriately reduced the power setting to medium to definitively scale any remaining calculus and optimize the debridement of biofilm from the root surfaces (Figures 8.7–8.9). Remember that a medium power setting is preferred over a low power setting for debridement, as medium power produces the greatest amount of cavitation without inherently over-instrumenting the root surface (Chapter 3).

The "correct" site-specific curved tip (right or left), that is, the configuration indicated for the treatment site, can be easily identified from the occlusal perspective (Figure 8.7a), as the contra-angle of the tip will bend toward the tooth, allowing for vertical adaptation of the active area, with the point of the tip directed away from the tooth.

The *right* curved tip was also utilized for debridement of the maxillary right palatal surfaces. As the tip crossed the ML line angle of #3 (FDI 16), the back of the tip adapted to the mesial surface (Figure 8.8a). Oblique strokes were implemented to advance the tip subgingivally and mesially across the mesial surface. Contact between the back of the tip and the mesial surface was maintained as the tip was transitioned to horizontal adaptation

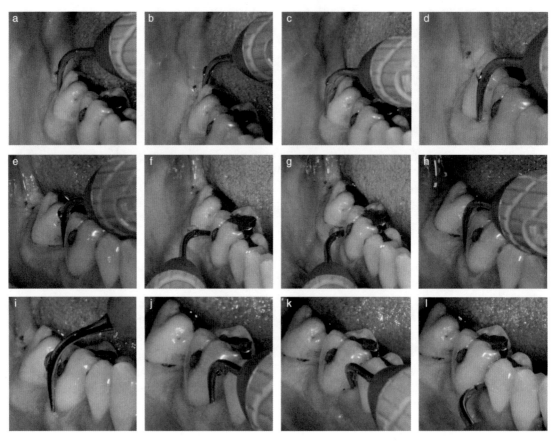

Figure 8.6 Proper adaptation and advancement of the tip is illustrated, beginning with (a) vertical adaptation at the DB line angle of #31 (FDI 47) and continuing, in sequential order, to (l) horizontal adaptation of the back of the tip to the mesial of #30 (FDI 46)

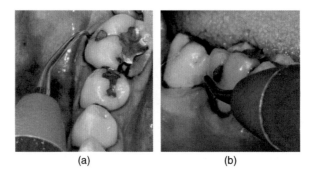

(a)   (b)

Figure 8.7 Vertical adaptation of the *right* curved tip at 0° to the buccal surface of #30 (FDI 46), as visualized from (a) occlusal and (b) buccal perspectives

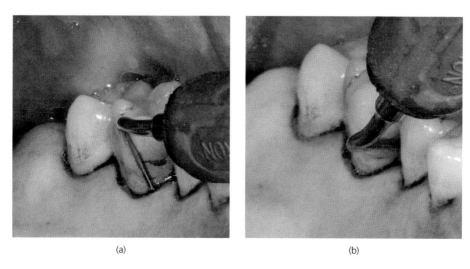

(a) (b)

Figure 8.8 Adaptation of the *right* curved tip in the maxillary right palatal sextant as visualized from the perspective of the right-handed clinician positioned at 12:00

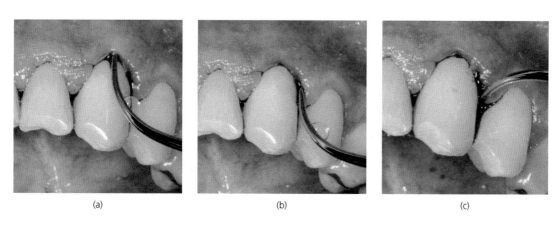

(a) (b) (c)

Figure 8.9 Advancement of a straight slim tip on the facial surface of #27 (FDI 43) from (a) midline to (b) the distal surface to (c) the distal interproximal space (from viewpoint of a right-handed clinician positioned at 12:00)

in the interproximal space (Figure 8.8b) and stroked vertically.

For debridement of the facial surfaces of the mandibular anterior sextant, either the *left* curved or a straight slim or ultraslim tip design can be utilized. In this case, the clinician opted to use a straight slim diameter tip.

As the mandibular anterior lingual sextant presented with the greatest amount of visible deposits, a comparison of the pretreatment and immediate posttreatment intraoral photographs of this area demonstrates the degree of deposit removal accomplished by ultrasonic instrumentation in this initial therapy case (Figure 8.10).

B. RE-EVALUATION

Three months post completion of initial therapy, a comparison of the initial and postdebridement probing depths was made (Figure 8.11), and intraoral photos were captured prior to commencing supportive

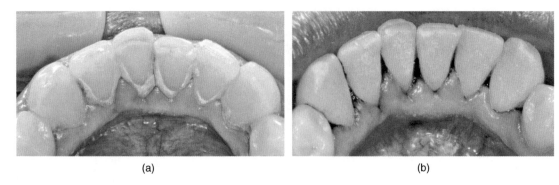

(a)   (b)

Figure 8.10 Comparison of the mandibular anterior lingual sextant (a) prior to and (b) immediately post initial nonsurgical ultrasonic periodontal debridement

PERIO CHART

Patient Name: Initial Periodontal Therapy Patient
    Patient ID:
    Exam Date: Re-evaluation

	1	2	3	4	5	6	7	8	9	10	11	12	13	14	15	16
MOB																
PD		3 3 3	3 2 4	3 1 3	3 1 3	3 2 2	2 2 3	3 2 3	3 2 3	3 2 3	3 1 3	3 2 3	3 2 3	3 2 4	5 2 2	
GM		2	1	1	2	1 0					1	1	1	1		
CAL		3 5 3	3 3 4	3 2 3	3 3 3	3 3 2	2 2 3	3 2 3	3 2 3	3 2 3	3 2 3	3 3 3	3 3 3	3 3 4	5 2 2	
MGJ																
PD (Ling)		4 2 5	5 2 4	4 2 3	3 2 3	3 2 3	2 2 2	2 2 2	2 2 2	2 2 2	2 2 3	3 2 3	3 2 3	4 3 4	5 3 3	
GM		2 1	1											1		
CAL		4 4 6	5 3 4	4 2 3	3 2 3	3 2 3	2 2 2	2 2 2	2 2 2	2 2 2	2 2 3	3 2 3	3 2 3	4 4 4	5 3 3	
MGJ																
Tooth	1	2	3	4	5	6	7	8	9	10	11	12	13	14	15	16

	32	31	30	29	28	27	26	25	24	23	22	21	20	19	18	17
MOB																
PD		3 2 3	4 2 4	4 2 4	4 2 3	3 2 2	2 2 2	2 1 2	2 1 2	2 1 3	3 1 3	3 2 3	3 2 4	4 3 4	4 3 5	
GM		1												1	1	
CAL		4 2 3	4 2 4	4 2 4	4 2 3	3 2 2	2 2 2	2 1 2	2 1 2	2 1 3	3 1 3	3 2 3	3 3 4	4 4 4	4 4 5	
MGJ																
PD (Bcl)		3 2 3	4 2 4	4 2 2	3 1 3	2 1 2	2 1 2	2 2 2	3 2 2	2 1 2	2 1 2	3 2 3	3 2 3	3 2 4	4 2 6	
GM																
CAL		3 2 3	4 2 4	4 2 2	3 1 3	2 1 2	2 1 2	2 2 2	3 2 2	2 1 2	2 1 2	3 2 3	3 2 3	3 2 4	4 2 6	
MGJ																
Tooth	32	31	30	29	28	27	26	25	24	23	22	21	20	19	18	17

Figure 8.11 Periodontal charting at reevaluation

ultrasonic instrumentation in these sextants (Figure 8.12).

Clinical Examination

– Resolution of inflammation was noted in numerous areas.

– Reduction of probing depths, which resulted in more accessible sites posteriorly was noted.

– Accumulation of soft debris and stain in isolated areas was used to determine areas where daily hygiene is inadequate.

C. SUPPORTIVE PERIODONTAL THERAPY (SPT)

Although calculus and stain were evident in some areas (Figure 8.12), the slight-moderate amount of calculus that formed could be efficiently removed concurrent with the disruption/removal of biofilm using debridement stage operational variables. Hence, the clinician executed all supportive periodontal instrumentation at a medium power setting utilizing curved slim and straight ultra-slim tips.

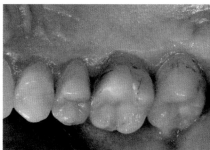
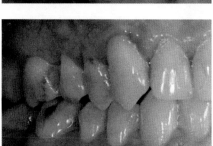
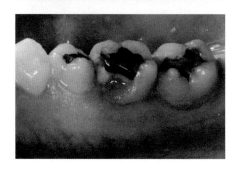

Initial Therapy Patient

3 Month Post-Op Photos

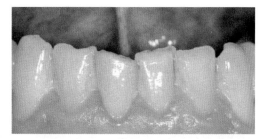
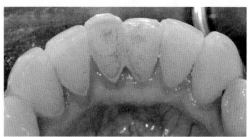

CASE A: INITIAL AND SUPPORTIVE PERIODONTAL THERAPY

Figure 8.12 Intraoral views of sextants 1, 5 and 6 at reevaluation

CASE STUDIES IN ULTRASONIC DEBRIDEMENT

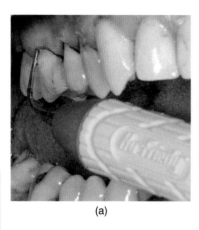

(a)

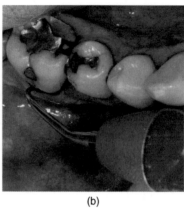

(b)

To reduce the frequency of changing tips, and thereby increasing the efficiency of instrumentation, the maxillary right buccal and mandibular right lingual sextants were first treated using the *left* curved insert (Figure 8.13a). The clinician then switched to the *right* curved tip to debride the mandibular right buccal (Figure 8.13b) and maxillary right palatal sextants.

Figure 8.13 Correct utilization and adaptation of (a) the left curved slim tip in the maxillary right buccal sextant and (b) the right curved slim tip in the mandibular right buccal sextant

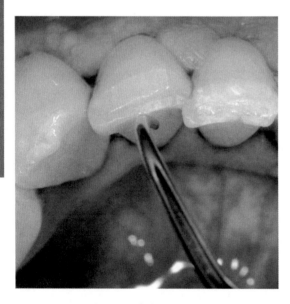

Before replacing the right curved tip, the clinician moved to the mandibular anterior lingual sextant to take advantage of the curvature of the right tip to remove stain and light deposits from the lingual fossa. Adapting the convex back of the curved tip to the concave fossa maximized contact and improved the efficiency of deposit removal in this area.

Figure 8.14 Utilization of the right curved tip in the mandibular anterior lingual sextant. Note how the convex back of the curved tip conforms to the concavity of the lingual surface of #23 (FDI 32)

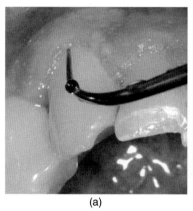 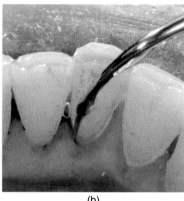

(a)   (b)

Figure 8.15 Adaptation of an ultraslim tip in (a) the facial sulcus of #22 (FDI 33) and (b) the lingual sulcus of #24 (FDI 31)

With the clinician already positioned for debridement of the mandibular anterior sextant, the right curved tip was replaced with a straight, ultraslim tip. The ultraslim diameter was preferred over the slim diameter for this area because of its more narrow diameter, which facilitated access into the shallow sulci and around the tight contacts, yet still produced sufficient amplitude at medium power to efficiently disrupt the biofilm and remove the slight-moderate calculus and stain present.

This case illustrates:

- Clinical application of the principles of ultrasonic instrumentation technique and sequencing

- Execution of ultrasonic instrumentation in two stages

- Appropriate selection of tip design and operational variables for each stage of instrumentation

- The process used to accomplish thorough removal of deposits utilizing only ultrasonic instrumentation

- The need for a variety of tip designs in order to implement effective ultrasonic instrumentation.

CASE A: INITIAL AND SUPPORTIVE PERIODONTAL THERAPY

CASE B: PREVENTIVE DEBRIDEMENT (ADULT PROPHYLAXIS) PATIENT

Presentation

- This 24-year-old Caucasian male presented for his routine (every 6–9 months) dental examination and cleaning.

Medical history

- The patient is a nonuser of tobacco, 6′ 0″ (1.83 m), weight 180 lbs (81.6 kg). BMI = 24.4 (normal weight). Patient takes no medication. Third molars were removed at age 18.

PERIO CHART

Patient Name: Adult Prophylaxis Patient
Patient ID:
Exam Date: Baseline

Tooth	1	2	3	4	5	6	7	8	9	10	11	12	13	14	15	16
MOB																
PD		3 2 3	3 3 3	3 3 3	3 3 3	3 3 3	3 3 3	3 3 3	3 3 3	3 2 3	3 3 3	3 3 3	3 3 3	3 3 3	3 3 3	
GM																
CAL		3 2 3	3 3 3	3 3 3	3 3 3	3 3 3	3 3 3	3 3 3	3 3 3	3 2 3	3 3 3	3 3 3	3 3 3	3 3 3	3 3 3	
MGJ																
Bcl	○○○	●●●	●●●	●●●	●●●	●●●	●●●	●○●	●○●	●○●	●○●	●●●	●●●	●●●	●●●	○○○
FG																
Ling	○○○	●●●	●●●	●●●	●●●	●○●	●○●	○○○	○●●	●○○	○●●	●●●	●●●	●●●	●●●	○○○
PD		3 2 3	3 3 3	3 3 3	3 3 3	3 2 3	3 2 3	3 2 3	3 2 3	3 2 3	3 3 3	3 3 3	3 3 3	3 3 3	3 3 3	
GM																
CAL		3 3 3	3 3 3	3 3 3	3 3 3	3 2 3	3 2 3	3 2 3	3 2 3	3 2 3	3 3 3	3 3 3	3 3 3	3 3 3	3 3 3	
MGJ																

Tooth	32	31	30	29	28	27	26	25	24	23	22	21	20	19	18	17
MOB																
PD		3 2 3	3 2 3	3 2 3	3 2 3	3 2 2	2 2 2	2 2 2	2 2 2	2 2 2	2 2 2	3 3 2	3 3 2	3 3 3	3 3 3	
GM																
CAL		3 2 3	3 2 3	3 2 3	3 2 3	3 2 2	2 2 2	2 2 2	2 2 2	2 2 2	2 2 2	3 3 2	3 3 2	3 3 3	3 3 3	
MGJ																
Bcl	○○○	●●●	●●●	●●●	●●●	●●●	●●●	●●●	●●●	●●●	●●●	●●●	●●●	●●●	●●●	○○○
FG																
Ling	○○○	●●●	●●●	●●●	●●●	●●●	●●●	●●●	●●●	●●●	●●●	●●●	●●●	●●●	●●●	○○○
PD		3 3 3	3 3 3	3 2 3	3 3 3	3 2 2	2 2 2	2 2 2	3 2 3	3 2 2	2 2 2	3 3 3	3 3 3	3 3 3	3 3 3	
GM																
CAL		3 3 3	3 3 3	3 2 3	3 3 3	3 2 2	2 2 2	2 2 2	3 2 3	3 2 2	2 2 2	3 3 3	3 3 3	3 3 3	3 3 3	
MGJ																

Figure 8.16 Periodontal charting of the preventive debridement (adult prophylaxis) patient

Clinical examination

- Maintainable probing depths (≤ 3 mm) were noted throughout the mouth.

- Isolated areas of minimal soft deposit and isolated areas of minimal supragingival calcified debris were noted in posterior areas.

- Bleeding on probing (BOP) was noted in multiple areas.

Radiographic examination

- No evidence of bone resorption was noted.

- No evidence of calcified debris was noted.

- Radiolucency consistent with incipient carious activity was noted on multiple interproximal surfaces.

Diagnosis

- Generalized gingivitis.

Treatment planned

- Preventive debridement (Adult prophylaxis)

- Prescribed daily home use of a CPP-ACP (casein phosphopeptide-amorphous calcium phosphate) product for remineralization

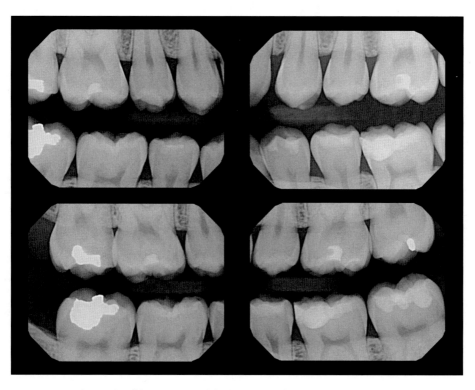

Adult Prophylaxis Patient
BWX

Figure 8.17 Bitewing radiographs of the preventive debridement (adult prophylaxis) patient

CASE B: PREVENTIVE DEBRIDEMENT (ADULT PROPHYLAXIS) PATIENT

Periodontal treatment provided

- Adult prophylaxis consisting of full-mouth ultrasonic debridement followed by coronal polishing.

Discussion

Although the patient's probing depths were within normal limits, inflammation and BOP were generalized throughout the dentition. Because no attachment loss had occurred, instrumentation to remove the biofilm and calculus is considered a preventive procedure and coded (according to ADA CDT codes) as an *adult prophylaxis*.

While the use of ultrasonic instrumentation during initial and supportive periodontal therapy for periodontitis is increasing, manual scaling (i.e., using hand instruments) continues to be the preferred method of instrumentation utilized by many clinicians for preventive procedures in patients such as this who have probing depths that are within normal limits.

Regardless of whether periodontal breakdown has or has not occurred, the etiology of the inflammation is the same – biofilm. Considering the advantages of cavitation and microstreaming in the disruption of biofilm combined with the availability of narrow diameter ultrasonic tips that can be easily inserted into shallow or tight sulci, these authors consider the use of

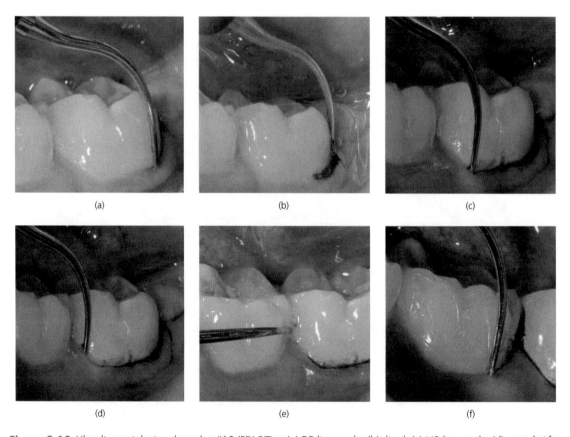

| (a) | (b) | (c) |
| (d) | (e) | (f) |

Figure 8.18 Ultraslim straight tip adapted at #18 (FDI 37) at (a) DB line angle; (b) distal; (c) MB line angle; (d) mesial. After transitioning to debride the mesial IP space, the tip is advanced to (e) the distal IP space of #19 (FDI 36) and then returned to vertical adaptation to continue debridement of (f) the buccal surface of #19 (FDI 36)

manual instruments for preventive debridement procedures to be illogical.

For this case, an ultraslim diameter tip oscillating in the range of medium power was utilized in all areas of the dentition. With probing depths within normal limits, the tip will only engage coronal anatomy, which typically is not highly contoured. Therefore, the straight tip can be adapted adequately to disrupt and reduce biofilm even at posterior sites. Figure 8.18 illustrates

proper adaptation around the mandibular left molars, commencing with insertion at #18 DB (FDI 37).

The ability of an ultraslim tip to easily debride shallow sulci and access areas of tight contact without causing significant distension of tissue, facilitating ultrasonic preventive debridement (ultrasonic prophylaxis), is most evident in this patient in the maxillary anterior palatal sextant.

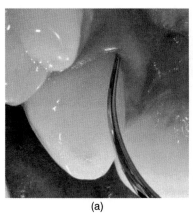 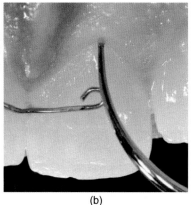

(a) (b)

The ultranarrow diameter allows the tip to slip between the free gingiva and the tooth surface with very minimal tissue distension.

Figure 8.19 Ultraslim tip adapted at mid-palatal of a maxillary cuspid and central incisor

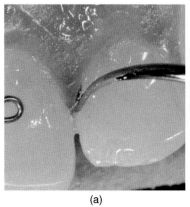 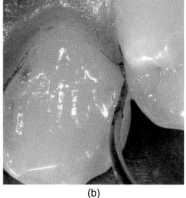

(a) (b)

Access of the active tip area to the interproximal surface is improved by the narrow dimension of the ultraslim tip.

Figure 8.20 Adaptation of an ultraslim tip at the interproximal surfaces of a maxillary lateral incisor and cuspid

CASE B: PREVENTIVE DEBRIDEMENT (ADULT PROPHYLAXIS) PATIENT

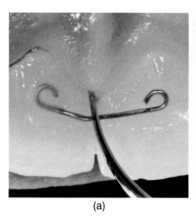 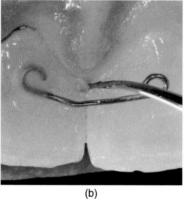

In areas of tight contact, accomplishing thorough debridement without supplemental use of a sickle scaler is only possible with the use of an ultraslim tip.

(a)   (b)

Figure 8.21 Accessibility of an ultraslim diameter tip to areas of tight contact

As the level of deposit presenting in this case was limited to biofilm and light calculus, instrumentation was implemented in one stage (debridement), using one tip design. Considering there was no need to change tips during instrumentation, the clinician improved the efficiency by implementing all instrumentation with only one change in operator position (Figure 8.22). Starting at the 12:00 position with the patient's head turned slightly to the right, the right-handed clinician chose to initiate instrumentation in the posterior region, beginning with the mandibular left buccal sextant. Maintaining operator and patient positions, instrumentation then advanced consecutively to the mandibular right lingual, maxillary left buccal, and maxillary right palatal sextants.

After instructing the patient to turn his head back to center, debridement of the mandibular and maxillary anterior sextants, both facial and lingual/palatal, was also executed from the 12:00 position.

Moving to the 8:00 position with the patient's head turned slightly left, the clinician completed debridement of the remaining sextants: maxillary right buccal and left palatal, and mandibular right buccal and left lingual.

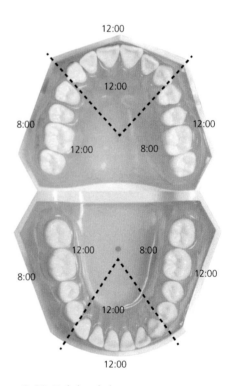

Figure 8.22 Right-handed operator positions utilized for efficient execution of preventive ultrasonic debridement instrumentation

This case illustrates:

- Application of ultrasonic instrumentation to preventive debridement procedures.

- Effectiveness of an ultraslim tip in accessing the anatomy of shallow sulci and tight contacts.

- Efficient execution of debridement stage instrumentation requiring only one change to operator position.

CASE B: PREVENTIVE DEBRIDEMENT (ADULT PROPHYLAXIS) PATIENT

CASE C: SURGICAL DEBRIDEMENT THERAPY

Presentation

This 47-year-old Caucasian male was referred for periodontal treatment from a private general dentistry practice. Initial periodontal therapy was completed in March. At the June supportive periodontal therapy appointment, reevaluation indicated the need for surgical debridement of the maxillary right quadrant.

Medical history

- The patient's height and weight are 5′10″ (1.78 m) and 190 pounds (86.2 kg). Body mass index (BMI) = 27.3 (overweight).

- Vital signs
  - BP 119/75 mm Hg
  - Pulse 65 bpm – regular

- The patient reports smoking slightly less than a half a pack (< 10 cigarettes) per day for the past five years.

- The patient is currently under medical care for high blood pressure and depression, both being treated with medication. The patient reports that his physician reevaluates his blood pressure control every three months.

- Surgery for diverticulitis ~5–7 years ago (2006–2008).

- Type II Diabetes controlled with diet and exercise; monitors glucose levels 2x/day; glucose levels usually range from 130–170 mg/dL. Most recent HbA1c (1 month ago) was 6.8%.

- Other: Patient reports limited mobility in arms; hearing issues in left ear.

- Medications:
  - NSAID, daily in the morning
  - Hydrochlorothiazide, daily for hypertension
  - SSRI (selective serotonin reuptake inhibitor), daily for depression
  - Simvastatin, daily for cholesterol reduction
  - Clonazepam, 3x/day for anxiety

- Allergies: Penicillin

- Physical status: ASA class II

Radiographic examination

- Advanced horizontal bone loss was noted at maxillary posterior areas and at tooth #7 (FDI 12), which is also root-filled.

- Calcified deposits were noted at #10 (FDI 22) distal; # 31 (FDI 47) mesial; and #18 (FDI 37) mesial.

- Retained primary tooth noted in place of tooth #29 (FDI 45).

- Less than ideal marginal contour of crown noted at #7 (FDI 12).

Clinical examination

- Initial probing depths (Figure 8.24) correlated with the radiographic appearance with deepened pocketing noted at maxillary posterior areas and isolated maxillary anterior areas

- Three months post initial periodontal therapy (Figure 8.25), persistence of inflammation was noted in several areas along with no significant reduction in probing depth. The depth and morphology of the persistent pockets (along with the lack of response to therapy) suggested that adequate debridement would not be possible without surgical access.

- Isolated areas of interproximal soft deposits were noted

- Isolated areas of bleeding on probing were noted.

Surgical Debridement Therapy Patient
Pre-treatment FMX

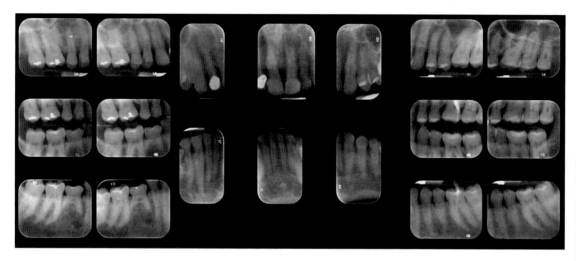

Figure 8.23 Pretreatment radiographs of a surgical debridement therapy patient

Risk assessment and diagnosis

- Risk factors for periodontal disease included tobacco use and diabetes. Potential link between being overweight and an increased risk for periodontal disease was discussed with the patient.

- Advised patient of potential interaction between cardiovascular disease, diabetes, and chronic periodontal disease.

- Diagnosis: Generalized chronic periodontitis

Periodontal treatment provided

Patient presented for surgical debridement and bone regeneration in maxillary right quadrant.

- A total of 216mg of 4% articaine w/0.054 mg epinephrine (three 1.8 ml cartridges w/1:100:000 epinephrine) was infiltrated throughout to anesthetize the quadrant.

- A full thickness mucoperiosteal flap was elevated to permit access to subgingival root surfaces and the alveolar crestal bone. Granulation tissue was surgically removed using a curet, and ultrasonic debridement of root surfaces was performed. Alveolar crestal bone was recontoured to create physiological contour. Cortical bone was perforated via #2 round bur with copious sterile water irrigation at tooth #3 (FDI 16) mesial. Reconstituted demineralized, freeze-dried bone was placed into the vertical bone defect at #3 (FDI 16) mesial. Interrupted 5-0 vicryl sutures were placed to reposition the flaps. Written and verbal postoperation instructions and pain prescription for Vicodin (acetaminophen and hydrocodone) were provided to patient.

Discussion

After reflecting the flap, the right and left curved tips and a straight furcation ball tip were utilized at a medium power setting to debride the exposed root surfaces. The surgical flap

CASE STUDIES IN ULTRASONIC DEBRIDEMENT

Surgical Debridement Patient   Comprehensive Periodontal Exam   Baseline

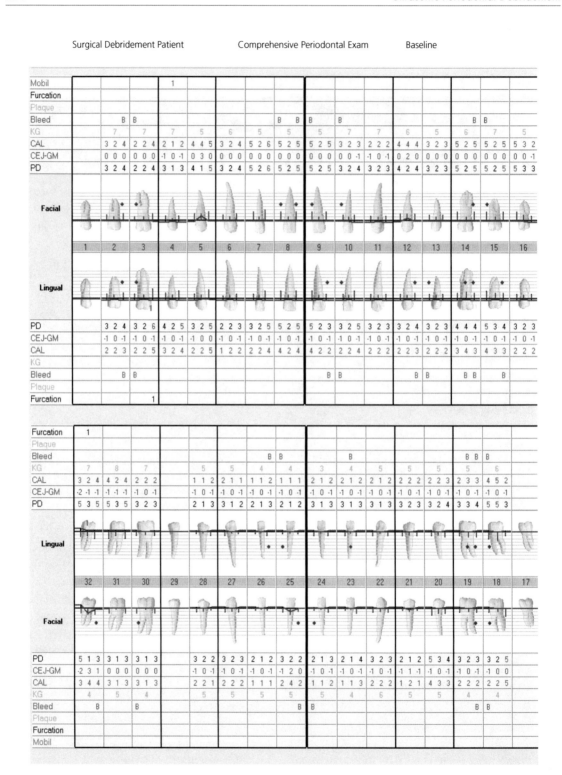

Figure 8.24 Pre-initial periodontal therapy charting of the surgical debridement patient

Surgical Debridement Patient   3 month Re-evaluation Exam

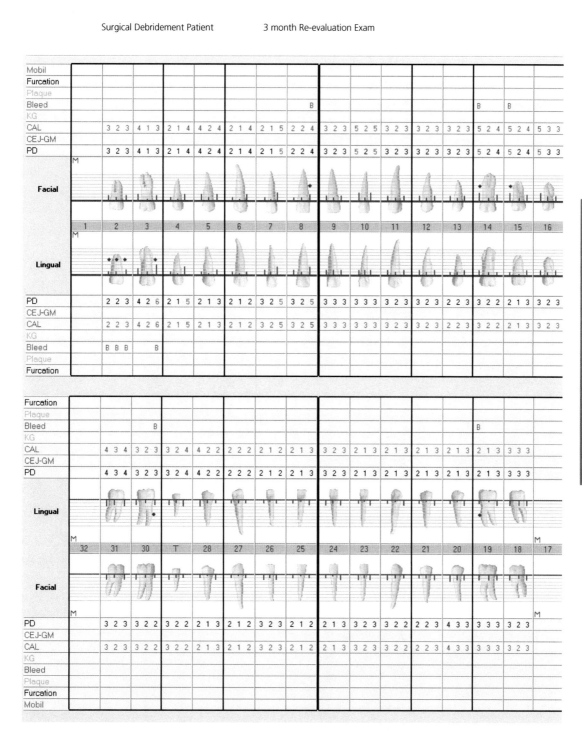

| | | 1 | 2 | 3 | 4 | 5 | 6 | 7 | 8 | 9 | 10 | 11 | 12 | 13 | 14 | 15 | 16 |

Facial / Lingual charting (upper arch):

	1	2	3	4	5	6	7	8	9	10	11	12	13	14	15	16
Mobil																
Furcation																
Plaque																
Bleed								B						B	B	
KG																
CAL		3 2 3	4 1 3	2 1 4	4 2 4	2 1 4	2 1 5	2 2 4	3 2 3	5 2 5	3 2 3	3 2 3	3 2 3	5 2 4	5 2 4	5 3 3
CEJ-GM																
PD		3 2 3	4 1 3	2 1 4	4 2 4	2 1 4	2 1 5	2 2 4	3 2 3	5 2 5	3 2 3	3 2 3	3 2 3	5 2 4	5 2 4	5 3 3
PD		2 2 3	4 2 6	2 1 5	2 1 3	2 1 2	3 2 5	3 2 5	3 3 3	3 3 3	3 2 3	3 2 3	2 2 3	3 2 2	2 1 3	3 2 3
CEJ-GM																
CAL		2 2 3	4 2 6	2 1 5	2 1 3	2 1 2	3 2 5	3 2 5	3 3 3	3 3 3	3 2 3	3 2 3	2 2 3	3 2 2	2 1 3	3 2 3
KG																
Bleed		B B B	B													
Plaque																
Furcation																

	32	31	30	T	28	27	26	25	24	23	22	21	20	19	18	17
Furcation																
Plaque																
Bleed			B											B		
KG																
CAL		4 3 4	3 2 3	3 2 4	4 2 2	2 2 2	2 1 2	2 1 3	3 2 3	2 1 3	2 1 3	2 1 3	2 1 3	2 1 3	3 3 3	
CEJ-GM																
PD		4 3 4	3 2 3	3 2 4	4 2 2	2 2 2	2 1 2	2 1 3	3 2 3	2 1 3	2 1 3	2 1 3	2 1 3	2 1 3	3 3 3	
PD		3 2 3	3 2 2	3 2 2	2 1 3	2 1 2	3 2 3	2 1 2	2 1 3	3 2 3	3 2 2	2 2 3	4 3 3	3 3 3	3 2 3	
CEJ-GM																
CAL		3 2 3	3 2 2	3 2 2	2 1 3	2 1 2	3 2 3	2 1 2	2 1 3	3 2 3	3 2 2	2 2 3	4 3 3	3 3 3	3 2 3	
KG																
Bleed																
Plaque																
Furcation																
Mobil																

Figure 8.25 Periodontal charting at the three month reevaluation

CASE C: SURGICAL DEBRIDEMENT THERAPY

procedure performed in this case provides an opportunity to observe the root anatomy encountered and compare the adaptation of the ultrasonic tip during closed debridement to that during open debridement.

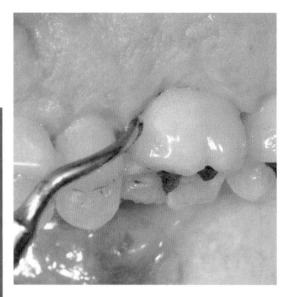

Figure 8.26

Adaptation of the *right curved* tip to the mesio-palatal root surface of #3 (FDI 16) during closed debridement shows how the length and curvature of this tip facilitates access to the root surface at the base of this 6 mm posterior interproximal pocket.

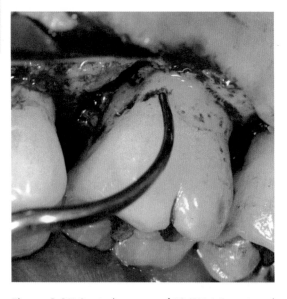

Figure 8.27 Surgical exposure of #3 (FDI 16) as viewed from the palatal aspect. Note the concavity on the mesial root surface and the residual calculus deposits on both the palatal and mesial surfaces

With surgical access, the contours of the mesial root surface and residual deposits are exposed.

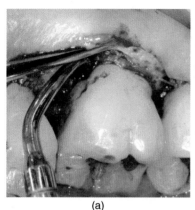 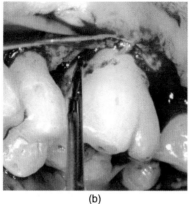

The flute of the mesial furcation was debrided using the back of the right curved tip (Figure 8.28a), as well as the ball-end of a straight furcation tip (Figure 8.24b). Observe the different methods of adaptation utilized with each tip.

(a)   (b)

Figure 8.28 Adaptation of (a) the right curved tip and (b) a straight furcation-ball tip to the flute of the mesial furcation #3 (FDI 16)

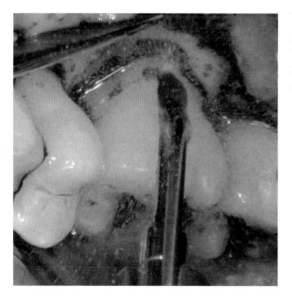

With the ball-end of the furcation tip adapted perpendicular to the mesial root surface, stroking was possible in multiple directions to efficiently remove residual calculus from the mesial root surface.

Figure 8.29 Utilization of the ball-end tip for the removal of residual calculus from the root surface of #3 (FDI 16)

CASE C: SURGICAL DEBRIDEMENT THERAPY

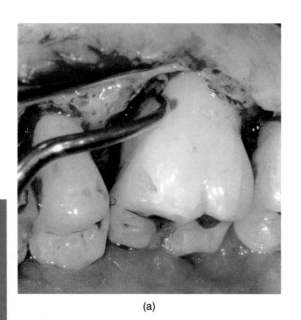

(a)

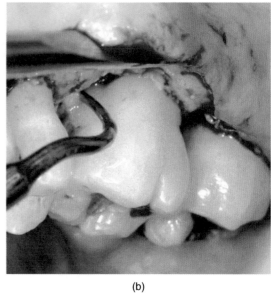

(b)

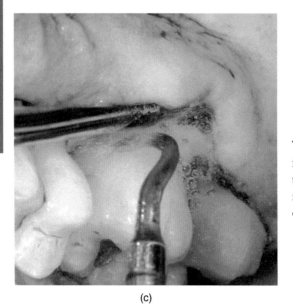

(c)

To complete debridement of the mesial root surface, the curvature of the right curved tip provided the degree of conformity needed to ensure that disruption of the biofilm on the concave surface was optimized (Figure 8.30).

Figure 8.30 Adaptation of the *right* curved tip at various points on the mesial root surface of #3 (FDI 16)

The capacity of the curved tip to innately conform to the concavities of root anatomy can also be observed on the mesial of tooth #5 (FDI 14), which demonstrates a marked mesial concavity (Figures 8.31 and 8.32).

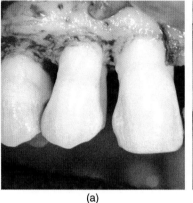 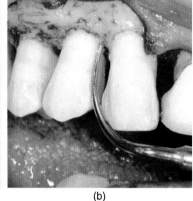

(a)   (b)

As the *left curved* tip is advanced across the MB line angle, vertical adaptation is maintained to allow the back of the tip to adapt to the mesial root surface.

Figure 8.31 (a) Surgical reflection of the buccal gingiva of #5 (FDI 14) exposes a pronounced mesial concavity; (b) adaptation of the convex back of the *left* curved tip to the mesial concavity

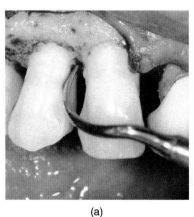 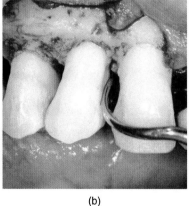

(a)   (b)

Note the degree of conformity attained as the back of the tip is advanced (a) apically and (b) lingually across the mesial surface using an oblique stroking pattern.

Figure 8.32

CASE C: SURGICAL DEBRIDEMENT THERAPY

This case illustrates:

- The application of ultrasonic instrumentation technique and sequencing to open debridement procedures.

- Appropriate utilization of a furcation-specific ultrasonic tip in a Grade I furcation defect.

- The innate capacity of the curved tips to conform to the concavities of root anatomy to the degree needed for optimal disruption of subgingival biofilm.

Glossary

Acceleration An increase in speed.

Acoustic Relating to sound, hearing, or the study of sound.

Acoustic microstreaming Small-scale, vigorous circulatory motion of fluid that occurs near objects in oscillatory motion.

Acoustic power The cumulative power exerted by the scaler tip as a result of the vibratory mechanism functioning synergistically with the forces of cavitation and microstreaming.

Active area The terminal 4 mm of the tip at which displacement amplitude is maximized; the portion of the tip which must adapt to the tooth surface for effective deposit removal.

Adaptation The position of the active area of the ultrasonic tip as it contacts the tooth surface.

Aerosol An airborne suspension of solid or liquid particles smaller than 50 μm in size.

Aerosolization The conversion of water emitted at the tip into a fine spray or mist resulting from a high power setting.

Angulation The geometric relationship between the active area of the ultrasonic tip and the tooth surface to be treated; ranges between 0° and 15°, keeping as close to 0° as possible and never exceeding 15°.

Auto-tuned Term used in reference to ultrasonic scaling units operating at a locked resonate frequency.

Bi-directional Movement of the tip in two opposing directions, such as forward-backward and upward-downward.

Biofilm A composition of microbial cells encased within a matrix of extracellular polymeric substances such as polysaccharides, proteins and nucleic acids; commonly referred to as *plaque*.

Cavitation The formation and subsequent implosion of pulsating cavities in a flowing liquid that is the result of forces acting upon the liquid.

Cross arch fulcrum Intraoral fulcrum established in the same arch, but opposite quadrant, as the treatment site.

Cupping retraction Retraction of the lip or cheek by pulling out, then up/down (lips) or out (cheek) in an attempt to contain the aerosol intraorally.

Debridement Instrumentation performed to disrupt and remove the subgingival biofilm and calculus, but without intentional removal of cementum; also referred to as *root surface debridement*.

Digital activation Activation of the working stroke by flexing of thumb, index, and middle fingers.

Displacement amplitude The amount of movement in a particular direction, as measured in microns (μm); measurement of how far the oscillating scaler tip is displaced in one direction from a position of zero movement.

Ecologic plaque hypothesis Theory which proposed that both the total amount of dental plaque and the specific microbial composition of plaque may contribute to the progression of periodontitis.

Elliptical stroke pattern Tip moves longitudinally and transversely (laterally) in the shape of an oval or ellipse.

Ultrasonic Periodontal Debridement: Theory and Technique, First Edition. Marie D. George, Timothy G. Donley and Philip M. Preshaw.
© 2014 John Wiley & Sons, Inc. Published 2014 by John Wiley & Sons, Inc.

Endotoxin Toxic substances within bacterial cells that are released upon cell death and which induce the inflammatory response which initiates and perpetuates breakdown of the periodontium; also referred to as *lipopolysaccharide.*

Equally-distributed The movement of the tip in each direction being equal in length; forward motion is no longer than backward motion.

Erasing motion Movement of the tip similar to erasing pencil mark from a piece of paper, characterized by bi-directional, equally distributed, short, over-lapping, and constant strokes.

Extraoral fulcrum Fulcrum established on an extraoral surface, such as the cheek or border of the mandible.

Frequency The rate at which something occurs or is repeated within a specific period of time; measured in *hertz* (Hz).

Frictional heating Increase in temperature resulting from two objects rubbing against each other when one or both objects are moving.

Fulcrum The point of stabilization during ultrasonic instrumentation; typically established distant to the treatment site.

Hertz (Hz) The standard unit of measurement of frequency; equivalent to 1 cycle per second.

High-volume evacuation (HVE) Removal of up to 100 cubic feet of air per minute; typically requires a large (>8 mm) bore (also referred to as *high volume aspiration*).

Horizontal adaptation Adaptation of the tip perpendicular to the long axis of the tooth so that the back or face of the tip contacts the treatment surface; same as *perpendicular adaptation.*

Horizontal stroke Movement of the tip in a left-right direction; utilized when the tip is in vertical adaptation.

Insertion The act of moving the ultrasonic tip into the treatment site. For supragingival instrumentation, insertion begins at an outermost edge of the deposit; for subgingival instrumentation, insertion begins at the gingival margin.

Kilohertz (kHz) A unit of measurement of frequency equivalent to 1000 cycles per second.

Kinetic energy Energy created by motion.

Lateral pressure The application of slight pressure or force against the ultrasonic tip when in contact with the tooth surface: also called *lateral force.*

Layering of protective procedures The adding on of protective procedures, or layers, to minimize the risk of cross-contamination.

Linear stroke pattern Tip moves longitudinally forward and backward in one plane; no lateral movement.

Lipopolysaccharide (LPS) A component of the outer cell wall of Gram-negative bacteria which invokes inflammatory responses in higher order species (often referred to as *endotoxin*).

Loaded Refers to a tip that is adapted against a tooth.

Magnetostriction A change in a material's physical dimensions in response to changing the magnetization of the material.

Manual-tuned Term used in reference to ultrasonic scaling units which allow adjustment of the operating frequency.

Minimum effective power The lowest level of power at which effective removal of the deposit can be achieved.

Newton (N) Standard unit of measurement of force.

Newton's Second Law of Motion This law states that the net force (F) of an object is a product of the object's mass (m) multiplied by its acceleration (a).

Nonspecific plaque hypothesis Theory which proposed that periodontal disease and caries resulted from harmful substances produced by the entire plaque mass, and that the main determinant of risk for disease was the amount of plaque present.

Oblique adaptation Adaptation of the tip oblique to the long axis of the tooth; method of adaptation used during manual instrumentation.

Oblique stroke Movement of the tip in a diagonal direction; utilized on interproximal root surface when the tip is in vertical orientation.

Opposite arch fulcrum Intraoral fulcrum established on the arch opposing the treatment site.

Oscillate To move forward and backward.

Parallel adaptation Adaptation of the tip parallel to the long axis of the tooth, with the point of the tip directed apically, toward the base of the pocket. Same as *vertical adaptation.*

Pellicle An organic material that coats all hard and soft surfaces in the oral cavity and functions as an adhesion site for bacteria.

Pen grasp The recommended grasp for holding an ultrasonic or sonic instrument, as it facilitates digital activation.

Perpendicular adaptation Adaptation of the tip perpendicular to the long axis of the tooth so that the back or face of the tip contacts the treatment surface. Same as *horizontal adaptation.*

Piezoelectric Materials which undergo dimensional changes when subjected to an electrical field.

Point of adaptation Site on the tooth surface where instrumentation commences; in ultrasonic instrumentation, points of adaptation are only utilized on the first tooth of the treatment area to initiate the instrumentation sequence.

Power setting The amount of electrical power input to the transducer; arbitrarily measured on a linear scale from low to high.

Quadrant One fourth of the dentition: there are four quadrants (upper right, lower right, upper left, lower left)

Resonant frequency A natural frequency of vibration determined by the physical parameters of the vibrating object.

Root planing Instrumentation performed to remove subgingival calculus and what was thought to be contaminated cementum from the root surface.

Root surface debridement (RSD) A light-touch, gentler form of instrumentation to remove and disrupt biofilm, yet with preservation of the cementum.

Scaling Instrumentation performed to remove or reduce both supragingival and subgingival calculus deposits.

Sextant One sixth of the dentition; there are two anterior sextants and four posterior sextants.

Sonic Sound waves having a frequency that is audible to the human ear.

Sonic scaler Air driven scaling device with an operating frequency in the sonic range, typically 16 kHz.

Splatter An airborne suspension of solid or liquid particles larger than 50 μm in size.

Split fulcrum Intraoral fulcrum established in same quadrant as treatment site, but with the middle finger having no contact or altered contact with the ring finger.

Stroke pattern The pattern of oscillation produced by an ultrasonic tip.

Tactile sensitivity The ability to distinguish tooth irregularities through the sense of touch from vibrations that are transmitted from the tip of an instrument to nerve endings in the fingers holding the instrument.

Tapping stroke Utilized only on supragingival calculus; point of the tip is gently "tapped" against calculus causing it to fracture.

Tip diameter Width of the tip in the active area.

Tip geometry The number of planes that the shank of the tip crosses; designated as either straight or curved.

Tip profile The number of bends in the shank of a tip.

Tip shape The shape of the active area of a tip in cross section, typically designed as either rectangular or circular.

Transducer A device that converts one type of energy into another.

Transitions Changes in adaptation made to advance the tip through the treatment area in a sequence that optimizes use of all surfaces of the tip.

Ultrasonic Sound (acoustic) energy having a frequency greater than 20 kHz, above the range audible to the human ear.

Unloaded The oscillation of a tip in air; not adapted against the tooth.

Vertical adaptation Adaptation of the tip parallel to the long axis of the tooth, with the point of the tip directed apically, toward the base of the pocket; same as *parallel adaptation*.

Vertical stroke Movement of the tip in an up-down direction; utilized when the tip is in horizontal adaptation.

Working stroke The movement of the tip activated by the clinician to advance the tip through the treatment site.

Index

Made in the USA
Coppell, TX
29 July 2021

59556528R00140